The Asian Diet

Also by Diana My Tran

The Vietnamese Cookbook

Contents

Foreword

The Asian Diet offers the more than 100 million overweight Americans a delicious and satisfying alternative to our high-fat, high-calorie eating habits. It is based on the flavorful wizardry of an outstanding Vietnamese chef who understands two of the world's finest culinary traditions—French and Asian. She is joined by a fine nutritionist, a person who maximizes nutritional delivery while minimizing calories. You will find these recipes satisfying because they are delicious and flavorful and because they cleverly rely on special Vietnamese sauces and herbs. You will also find that the Asian diet is consistent with the latest nutritional thinking, which emphasizes wonderful ways to cook and serve the fruits, vegetables, rice, and fish we all need to maximize health benefits while losing weight and maintaining a healthy active lifestyle.

Why We Need the Asian Diet

Well over half of the American adult population is considered overweight, according to government data. Millions of these people are suffering from illnesses they could avoid if they reduced their body fat and increased their physical activity. For years, Americans have been warned about the health risks associated with excess fat and the huge expense of treating diseases that are more common among the overly fat. All of this talk is getting us nowhere. The problem is worsening with every passing year, and now even teenagers and small children are suffering skyrocketing rates of obesity and diabetes.

In 1994, former U.S. Surgeon General C. Everett Koop founded a nonprofit organization—Shape Up America!—whose mission is to provide sound information on weight management through healthy eating and increased physical activity. The following year, Dr. Koop asked me to assume the leadership of Shape Up America! because of my scientific background and training in weight management program development. What came as a surprise to Dr. Koop, and what few people know, is that my personal history has been shaped by my own struggles with excess fat. I also learned that Dr. Koop was working very hard to manage his weight to delay knee surgery as long as possible. The health consequences of excess fat were a personal issue for both of us.

My Diet History

While I did not try every fad diet ever published to handle my weight problem, I confess I did try one or two. While I struggled, I watched slim people eat normal meals, and I realized that fad dieting was a silly and self-stigmatizing approach to the problem. Finally, I went to one commercial program with a good reputation for educating people with weight problems. I showed up faithfully each week, for many months, and I did everything required. I kept detailed records of what I ate, I kept track of my feelings when I ate, and I was a serious and committed student of weight loss. And I succeeded. I lost weight slowly, and I reached my goal weight. I was jubilant. I was a star, and I bought a new outfit to show off my new figure. But shortly thereafter, like millions of other dieters, I started to regain the weight. I hadn't really figured it out. As it turns out, I had a lot more to learn.

The Epiphany

Through this experience, I realized how little I knew about food and how to manage my behavior to ensure long-term success. I was amazed to learn that weight management required an active commitment—a daily rededication to exercise and daily diet vigilance.

It was my sister who put it into words for me. She explained to me how she realizes now she can never again eat the way she did as a kid—mindlessly, thoughtlessly—without any concern about weight. Now and forever, she sighed, she must pay attention to everything she puts in her mouth. I rebelled against this; I thought it sounded like slavery. But the day came when I realized that it was true for me, too. Failure to grasp this reality had been the cause of my weight regain. This was my epiphany.

Even this meaningful discovery was not enough. I was born with a robust appetite. My family is from farming stock and farmers have big appetites. I was pitted against my natural inclination to eat a lot of food. I eventually came to realize that I may have a farmer's appetite, but I don't work on a farm. I worked at a desk and would probably work at a desk for the rest of my life. How was I going to live in the 21st century with a set of 19th-century genes and not get fat?

Energy Balance—What Is It? How Does It Relate to My Life?

The solution that worked for me was energy balance. Energy balance is simple: It is calorie balance—calories in balanced by calories out. Food provides the calories in, and exercise and other voluntary activity are the calories out. I could live with my big appetite if I balanced it with plenty of physical activity. An understanding of energy (or calorie) balance is critical for people who like to eat, but don't want to get fat. We have to focus on delicious, flavor-packed food that delivers a delightful eating experience while delivering as few calories as possible. And we have to exercise daily.

Portion Sizes Are the Key to Weight Loss

In *The Asian Diet*, as in all successful diets, the portion sizes are your key to calorie management. If a recipe serves four people, and only two of you are sitting down to dinner, stand ready with refrigerator containers. You will want to set aside the remaining two servings to enjoy on another day. If you pay close attention to portion control, calories will take care of themselves. This is accomplished almost effortlessly because of the heavy emphasis on vegetables that are naturally low in fat and high in fiber.

Exercise and Calorie Dilution— Scientific Breakthrough

Hunger and malnutrition were common in America at the beginning of the 20th century, and food fortification and government feeding programs played a key role in just about eliminating these problems. But by the end of the century, overeating and obesity replaced hunger and nutritional deficiency diseases as the leading nutritional problems. These problems will not be solved so easily. The good news is that breakthroughs in scientific research offer insights that will help us move in a healthier direction.

The first insight is that dieting does work—we can lose weight and we often do. What we are not good at is keeping the weight off. Why? Two reasons: 1) Most of us refuse to accept the truth: we have to be mindful of what we eat for the rest of our lives—day in and day out; and 2) Restricting calories may work for weight loss but it does not work to keep the weight off permanently; most studies show that increasing exercise is necessary to prevent weight regain.

There is hardly an American alive who has not dieted. We have a great deal of experience losing weight using both sound and unsound weight loss diets. Yet, as a nation, we suffer from a higher prevalence of overweight and obesity than ever. Why have repeated cycles of weight loss and regain become the American "weigh of life"? The reason is that few of us understand how to keep the pounds off. It was not until the past 10 years that we have begun to understand what it takes to prevent weight gain or regain after dieting. Although it may sound like heresy to say it, exercise is not as powerful as restricting food intake if your goal is weight loss. Study after study shows that a weight loss strategy that relies strictly on exercise produces only four to six pounds of weight loss. To lose weight, you have to learn how to manage food—learning proper portion control and consuming fewer calories—but exercise is absolutely critical for keeping the weight off. Few people successfully maintain weight loss if they refuse to exercise.

Walking is a perfectly acceptable and effective form of exercise. The only catch is, you have to do it every day for 30 minutes. This goal is not so difficult to achieve once you realize that three 10-minute walks are as good as one 30-minute walk. For many people, just 10,000 steps a day is what it takes for weight management. Expressed in calories, that is approximately 2,200 exercise calories a week for women and 2,500 exercise calories a week for men.

The next insight is that you can fool yourself into eating fewer calories if you know how to prepare or select meals that will dilute the calories while preserving good flavor. A satisfying and easy way to do this is to follow the menu plans presented in this book. They are flavorful and highly satisfy-

ing, and they deliver plenty of food but minimize the calories. What could be easier?

Tracking Success

As a final thought, consider the bathroom scale as an inexpensive tool for monitoring your weight loss progress or your weight management success. Better yet, for a few dollars more, you can buy a body fat analyzer. A body fat analyzer will allow you to stop obsessing over your weight and place your focus where it belongs—on your body fat content. For good health, it's not your weight that counts; it's the proportion of fat and muscle in your body. Have you ever undertaken an exercise program and, after eight weeks, were demoralized to discover that all of your exercise efforts resulted in weight gain? If you had a body fat analyzer, you would have learned that over that eight-week period your body fat decreased, your muscle strength and tone increased, and your health status improved! You were successful without knowing it!

Even if weight management is not a goal for you, the beauty and flavor of the recipes and menu plans in *The Asian Diet* are reason enough to want to own the book and use it regularly. You will discover that this is one of the most delightful ways to increase your consumption of foods like vegetables and fish—rich sources of antioxidants and other nutrients that offer cancer protection and other benefits to your health. This book is a sincere effort to delight you and, at the same time, guide you toward a healthier way of eating. I wish you long life, good eating, and good health.

Barbara J. Moore, Ph.D.
President and CEO
Shape Up America!
www.shapeup.org

Acknowledgments

Years ago, all I could dream of was to own a small house and be settled comfortably in this country. I never thought of becoming an author and, hard to believe, this is my second book. I was once asked how I define success. I was not hesitant to say that success is a road that is always under construction. I will never satisfy all of my aspirations. I have found myself many times struggling up and down on that road. What kept me moving, despite numerous obstacles, was the motivation from my family and friends. They were always there, encouraging, supporting, cheering, loving, and, mostly, tolerating me unconditionally. I may never get to what so-called success is, but I already feel successful and proud to have friends who contribute so much to my life. I would like to send my deepest thanks and appreciations to:

My publisher, Kathleen Hughes—Once again you have given me not only a great opportunity, but also a strong feeling of confidence and accomplishment.

Dr. Barbara Moore, president of Shape-Up America!—Thank you for participating and sharing your valuable knowledge. I greatly appreciated it.

Dr. Idamarie Laquatra, my excellent nutritionist—I was blessed to have found you and worked with you. Your friendship and partnership will always be treasured.

Steve Raymer, my wonderful photographer—I thank you deeply for your exquisite talent in making both of my books so beautiful.

Suzanne St.Pierre, for your generosity and support—Thanks again for giving me a great party for *The Vietnamese Cookbook*. It made me feel very special.

Ann Yonkers, for all your kindness and willingness to help me throughout this project.

Ann Yick, for understanding and listening to all my problems.

To Neil and Sandra Willett Jackson, for such a wonderful friendship.

Mindy Weisel, for being a true friend.

All my customers at Diana's Couture and Bridal—I never would have become an author without the strong incentive and support all of you have given me.

To my family and friends, for the love and intensive support to make my dreams come true.

PART 1

Getting Slim the Asian Way

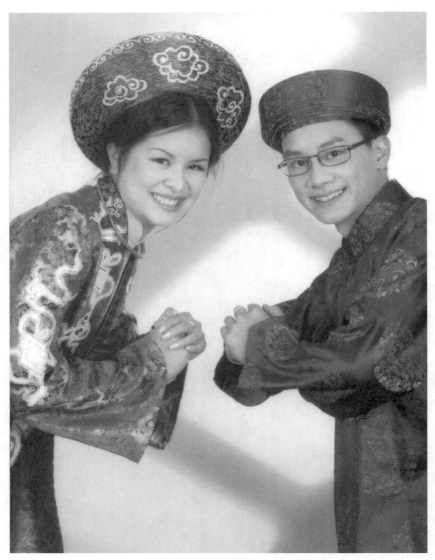

Vietnamese children in America have to adjust themselves to both Asian and Western cultures. Although born in America, John, 26, and Diana Tran, 19, still value Vietnamese traditions. They enjoy American food as well as Vietnamese food. They were proud to dress in their traditional Vietnamese outfits on our July 2001 family trip to Vietnam.

CHAPTER 1

"Why Asians Are Not Fat"

"Why aren't Asians fat? What is your daily diet?" People have asked me the same questions many times. My answer is unique and simple: I eat Vietnamese foods. My American clients were amazed with my reply. Vietnamese cuisine is an interesting blend of Asian and French techniques, seasonings, and flavors. I remember when I first came to this country in 1975; my American friends were still skeptical when I tried to introduce Vietnamese foods to them, but it did not take me long to convince them. Asian/Vietnamese cuisine is increasingly favored in America because of its healthy, authentic ingredients. The Asian diet is influenced by family traditions, eating patterns, and use of their most important ingredients, including rice, fish/seafood, abundant herbs and vegetables, fruits, and teas.

Family Traditions and Eating Patterns

Growing up in Vietnam, I remembered my family's tradition. Breakfast was often a bowl of fried rice and a cup of hot soybean milk or café au lait, or if we were on the run, a piece of French sandwich or sweet rice wrapped in a banana leaf. Dinner would be the most important meal of the day, the time for family to get together. All of us would sit down for the daily meal during which we would share our thoughts and ideas and our daily experiences and enjoy the company of our family. We also looked forward to the menu of the day, which would include dishes that we requested that morning. My father loved the freshly caught fish bought at the market and deliciously prepared by my sister. I particularly liked abundant fresh vegetables with terribly spicy sauce, more often my invention. We always had a big bowl of clear vegetable soup that we all shared. For dessert, our favorite was fresh fruit of the season.

Living in America, I still try to keep my family heritage alive, although it is much harder here because of the fast pace. Cooking a traditional Vietnamese dinner for my family of four can be a major effort after a long day at work. Our dinner usually starts at 8:30 at night. It is late to eat a heavy meal, so I prefer to serve more vegetables to help digestion before we go to bed. We don't have much time to talk to our children, so I try to get them to eat dinner with us as often as I can. My son, John, 26, has a busy schedule. If he cannot make it for dinner, I just save him his favorite dish. My daughter

Diana, 19, is a freshman at Marymount College and, to my surprise, is a traditional Vietnamese in the foods she prefers. She loves all the authentic Vietnamese dishes that most of the kids would hesitate to try. Her enjoyment is special to me because we can savor my specialty without a doubt together. Having the children home, John joking around, Diana helping with the chopping and cleaning, makes me feel very blessed. It actually relieves the stress and tension of a long day at work. Diana seems to like more vegetables than meat. John, on the other hand, loves steak once a week.

My husband likes fish, vegetables, and very little meat. He is thinking about becoming a vegetarian, so vegetables account for a large part of our daily diet. Often, I balance my diet with more vegetables and fish or seafood and just a moderate amount of meat, especially red meat. Over the years, I have created my own easier and healthier versions of Vietnamese dishes. It takes much less time to cook fish, shrimp, and vegetables than it does to cook meat. Once or twice a week, I have a meat or poultry dish to please my two Vietnamese/American children, and rice, of course, is essential.

My father always said "perfect rice" is the key to his meal. In the winter, I often cook a big pot of soup consommé and serve it with noodle and fresh herbs. It lasts my family two days and saves me some cooking time. Frequently, my family prefers rice. On the weekend, if I feel overworked, my kitchen is "closed for the day," and we go to our favorite restaurant. I don't try to diet or lose weight, but, thanks to our traditional foods, our diet seems to do the work.

Vietnamese cuisine is a combination of Chinese, Japanese, Korean, and Thai delicacies, and spices and seasonings play a critical role. Vietnamese serve a variety of sauces at every meal, and the most common major ingredients of the Asian diet are rice, vegetables, seafood/fish, pickles, and salads.

Important Ingredients of the Asian/Vietnamese Diet

Rice

Agriculture is a major industry in most Asian countries; in fact, Vietnam is one of the countries of Southeast Asia known for its vast rice fields. The Mekong Delta is the major rice basket of Southern Vietnam. Today, the region is one of Vietnam's best producers of rice crops, vegetables, and fruits. Rice, the foundation of the Asian diet, is eaten daily. It is a healthy and nutritious source of carbohydrates, vitamins, and minerals, contains less fat than wheat, and has no allergenic protein as wheat does, so rice allergies are rare. There are many varieties of rice, distinguished by their color and shape. Asians prefer white rice. Chinese like it dry and concentrate more on the entrées, while Vietnamese prefer it moist and fluffy.

White Rice: Whole-grain and white in color, this rice is a daily staple of the Asian/Vietnamese diet.

Brown Rice: Long-grain and unpolished, brown rice has more fiber than white rice and helps to reduce cholesterol. Asians believe eating brown rice can prevent cancer and other major diseases.

Black Rice: Black in color, this rice has a nutty taste, similar to wild rice, and is also a good source of fiber.

Glutinous Rice (also called sticky rice or sweet rice): This rice is white, long, short, or round-grained, and takes on a glutinous consistency when cooked.

Fish and Seafood

Fish and seafood play an important role in Asian diets; in most parts of Asia, they account for approximately 40 percent of people's daily supply of protein. In Asia, particularly Southeast Asia, fish and seafood are always available, freshly caught, in markets. In America, they sometimes can be found at fish markets and fresh or frozen in the local supermarket. Some fish and shrimp are also dried and eaten that way. Southeast Asians use fish to make fish sauce or paste, both of which are very common in Thai, Laotian, and Vietnamese cuisine.

Sauces

Fish sauce is a principal ingredient in South Asian cuisine. Asians use it straight from the bottle for cooking or as an ingredient in Sweet and Sour Fish Sauce. Fish sauce accompanies every meal in Vietnam.

Soy sauce is made from soybeans. Buddhist vegetarians use it for seasoning, and Japanese and Koreans use it in place of fish sauce.

Also made from soybeans, hoisin sauce differs from soy sauce in its slightly sweet taste and its thick, jamlike consistency. Chinese recipes often call for black soybean sauce.

Oyster sauce, a concentrated extract of oysters, is one of the main ingredients used in Asian cooking. It is especially favored in Chinese and Vietnamese sauté dishes.

Red vinegar is a popular Chinese condiment and an important influence in Vietnamese flavoring. Asians believe red vinegar helps to break down the fat in their diet, especially in meat dishes.

Hot pepper sauce, made from ground chili peppers, is used in any dish to add a hot, spicy taste. Thai chili peppers are among the hottest and spiciest peppers and are used mostly in spicy Thai dishes. It is also an important component of the Vietnamese sweet and sour fish sauce. Japanese prefer their food to be milder, and Koreans add dry ground red pepper to all preserved pickles, such as cucumber pickles and kimchee.

Spices

Characteristic of Southeast Asian cuisine is the interesting blend of spices and seasonings. Most Asians are familiar with five-spice powder, curry powder, black pepper, dry red pepper, star anise, and turmeric powder. Fresh lemongrass, garlic, dill, galanga, ginger, scallions, basil, chives, cilantro, culantro, and cayang, on other hand, are key elements in Vietnamese and Thai cooking.

Vegetables

Practically all Asians love vegetables, and they have similar techniques for preparing them. In Vietnam, one can find freshly picked produce in open-air markets, and Vietnamese cooking uses it abundantly, with only a small amount of meat. Vietnamese often eat vegetables raw, steamed, or stir-fried. Traditionally, they wrap the raw vegetables and herbs (lettuce, cucumber, green mustard, basil, cilantro, culantro, cayang, chives) and dip them in their favorite sauce, often the famous sweet and sour fish sauce. This is a Vietnamese-style salad. In addition, Vietnamese families often serve clear vegetable soup as part of every meal.

Fruit

Asians eat fruit for snacks and dessert. In America, Asian supermarkets carry a variety of tropical fruits, such as bananas, mangoes, papayas, tangerines, grapefruits, pineapple, longan (found in Vietnam and Thailand, this fruit tastes like lychee), and many seasonal fruits imported from Asia. Most of Vietnam's fruits come from the Mekong Delta.

Tea

Tea is a necessity in Asian families. In Vietnam, most people drink fresh green tea, and Koreans and Japanese generally prefer green tea. Other tea varieties are black, jasmine, chrysanthemum, and lotus. Thai iced tea, in particular, is popular in America. Vietnamese and Chinese drink hot tea after dinner; they believe tea takes away the fat in food and helps digestion. Adding ginger to tea is a good home remedy for colds and stomachaches, or just to give it an extra special flavor. Ancient Vietnamese and Chinese consider drinking tea to be an art and reflective of a philosophy. It helps to begin a conversation or a friendship, or drinkers simply enjoy its aroma.

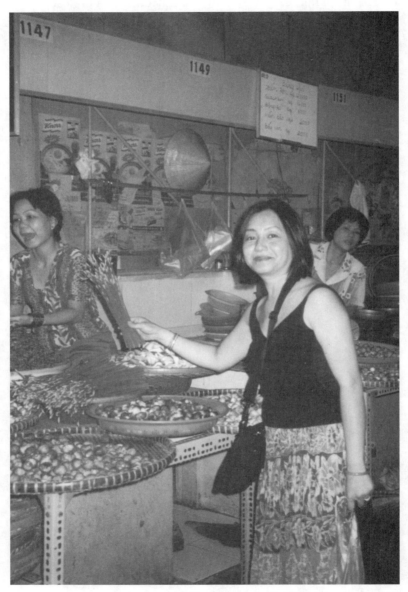

Here I am at the Ben Thanh market in Vietnam last July 2001. I found myself enjoying grocery shopping like it was years ago. I was particularly thrilled when I found a fresh bunch of Garlic Chives, which I use in some recipes in this book.

2 A **Nutritionist** Looks at the **Health Benefits** of Asian Cuisine

CHAPTER

The Asian diet is plant-based. Abundant fruits and vegetables grace the meals, and tofu is used in innovative and flavorful ways. A variety of seafood is prepared with tasty sauces, and meat, while present, is not the focal point of the meal. What are the benefits of eating this way?

The Good News about Fruits and Vegetables

The research linking fruit and vegetable consumption to protection against many diseases continues to grow. Specific components of fruits and vegetables are thought to confer benefits—for example, they are a great source of antioxidants, which protect the body from unstable oxygen by-products called free radicals. Free radicals are generated by normal body processes as well as by radiation or ultraviolet light, air pollutants, and cigarettes. They can damage genetic material, cell membranes, enzymes, and other cell components. Scientists have linked free radicals with many diseases and conditions, including cancer, heart disease, Parkinson's, cataracts, arthritis, diabetes, and even aging. Protective enzymes in our bodies are one line of defense to neutralize free radicals; antioxidants are another. Listed in the following table are antioxidant vitamins and their food sources.

Antioxidant	Food Source
vitamin E	wheat germ, vegetable oils
vitamin C	fruits and vegetables, especially broccoli, cantaloupe, citrus fruits, peppers, tomatoes, strawberries
beta-carotene (transformed to vitamin A in the body)	yellow fruits and vegetables and green, leafy vegetables, such as cantaloupe, peaches, apricots, carrots, sweet potatoes, spinach

Fruits and vegetables also contain naturally occurring substances called phytochemicals that appear to be quite effective in preventing and treating heart disease and cancer.

The table below lists a sampling of fruits and vegetables and the phytochemicals they contain. As you can see, a diet with plenty of fruits and vegetables provides good sources of phytochemicals. Eating fruits or vegetables is preferable to taking supplements containing the phytochemical, because the whole food provides a variety of beneficial substances. It is becoming evident that the substances in fruits and vegetables work together, like a team, to provide their healthful effects.

Food	Phytochemical
apples	pectin
blackberries, blueberries, cherries, cranberries, grapes, plums, raspberries, corn, red onions, red cabbage, sweet potatoes	anthocyanins
broccoli, cabbage, cauliflower	isothiocyanates
cabbage, broccoli, brussels sprouts	indole-3-carbinol
grapefruit, lemons, limes, oranges	limonoids
garlic	allyl compounds
tomatoes	lycopene

Here is more good news: fruits and vegetables are a great source of dietary fiber. Fiber is the part of plant foods that cannot be digested by the enzymes in our intestines. There are two different types of dietary fiber, soluble and insoluble. Soluble fiber forms a gel in water, and insoluble fiber gives plants their structure. Both provide benefits. Soluble fiber helps to stabilize blood sugar levels in people with diabetes and has been found to lower blood cholesterol, and insoluble fiber helps prevent and treat constipation. Fruits and vegetables contain both types of fiber.

The Tofu Story

What Is Tofu?

My two aunts in Vietnam are Buddhist vegetarians, and tofu is the main source of protein in their daily diet. When I was a little girl, I watched them preparing many tofu dishes and loved them all. I was taught to eat tofu in many different, creative ways.

Fried or raw, soft or firm, tofu became my favorite ingredient in cooking. In the Western diet, tofu is much less understood. I am often asked what tofu is, what it tastes like, and how to cook it. I'd like to share with you some of my aunts' tofu specialties, but first, it is helpful to learn more about tofu to be able to cook it and love it.

Tofu, made from soybean, comes in two categories: soft or silken tofu and firm tofu. Soft or silken tofu has a smooth, silky-soft consistency. It can be used raw, in soups, ginger syrup for dessert, or dips. Silken tofu does not stir-fry well. Firm tofu, on the other hand, is best fried, especially stir-fried with vegetables, and often replaces meat in vegetarian cooking. Raw tofu has a bland flavor, somewhat like cottage cheese, and must be cooked properly to be tasty. Both firm and silken tofu are now available in most grocery stores in the produce section. Tofu is like a dairy product; it is normally sold in plastic tubs, immersed in water, and should be refrigerated. Before using tofu, pour off the water, rinse, and pat dry. Silken and firm tofu often come inside foil packages, imported from Japan, and have a very long shelf life. Firm tofu is sold freshly made in Asian grocery stores.

What Are the Benefits of Tofu?

Soy protein is the only complete protein found in a plant. Low in calories and cholesterol-free, tofu can be an excellent calcium source if it is processed with calcium. Research on soybeans has demonstrated its benefit for reducing the risk of heart disease and cancer; eating soy protein can reduce heart disease risk by lowering blood cholesterol levels, which, if high, are a risk factor for heart disease. The U.S. government backs the health claim that consuming 25 grams or more of soy protein per day as part of a low-fat, low-cholesterol diet may reduce the risk of heart disease. Reaching the 25 grams per day is not difficult if you follow an Asian diet. Four and a half ounces of firm tofu contain 15 grams of soy protein, and one eight-ounce glass of soymilk contains 10 grams.

Soy also contains isoflavones, compounds that have weak estrogen-like activity. Isoflavones compete with estrogen in the body, which means they "tie up" places where estrogen would normally exert some negative effects. In countries where soy consumption is high, the incidence of breast, prostate, and uterine cancer is lower than in the United States. The lower incidence of the cancers may be related to isoflavones, but the research is not yet conclusive. Soy sources of isoflavones are soymilk, sprouts, soy flour, and tofu.

The Benefits of Fish

Many Asian recipes use different varieties of fish and shellfish, rich sources of omega-3 fatty acids, a class of polyunsaturated fatty acids. Current research indicates that omega-3 fatty acids protect the heart. They lower blood fats (triglycerides) and appear to reduce the chance of sudden cardiac death. Ocean fish containing the most omega-3s include sardines, salmon, mackerel, tuna, sablefish, and herring. Freshwater fish such as trout are also good sources.

Shellfish include clams, crab, lobster, mussels, oysters, scallops, and shrimp. Their primary nutritional benefit is their low level of saturated fat. Saturated fat increases blood cholesterol, and people have been advised to reduce their intake of foods that are high in saturated fat. For years, people with high blood cholesterol were advised to limit shellfish consumption or avoid shellfish completely because it was believed that these foods were too high in cholesterol. Newer methods for measuring the cholesterol in shellfish revealed that the older methods overestimated the amount of cholesterol. Shellfish and fish are now considered to be appropriate foods in a heart-healthy diet.

Meat: Out of the Spotlight

In many Asian recipes, meat does not take center stage but is more like a condiment added to the dish. While providing an excellent source of protein and iron, meat unfortunately is a major source of saturated fat. Because the Asian diet moderates the use of meat, the total amount of saturated fat is less than in most American diets.

Going Vegetarian

People choose a vegetarian lifestyle for many reasons, including personal philosophy, culture, religion, and health. There are different types of vegetarians, and each type excludes different animal products. A *vegan* does not eat any animal products at all. An *ovo-vegetarian* does not consume dairy products, meat, fish or poultry, but will eat eggs. A *lacto-vegetarian* eats dairy products but no eggs, meat, fish or poultry. A *lacto-ovo-vegetarian* eats eggs and dairy products, but no meat, fish, or poultry. "Semivegetarians" include people who don't eat red meat, but enjoy fish and poultry, and those who eat only small amounts of animal products. Asian cuisine can be adapted to fit any vegetarian lifestyle.

Healthy Foods Can Taste Great

Eating healthfully has suffered a bad reputation because some diets have been short on taste. People are not willing to sacrifice taste, even if they are concerned about their health. In fact, taste is the number one consideration when making food choices. The Asian diet includes cooking processes that preserve the fresh taste of the ingredients. Each dish is a delicious package that delivers the bonus of good nutrition.

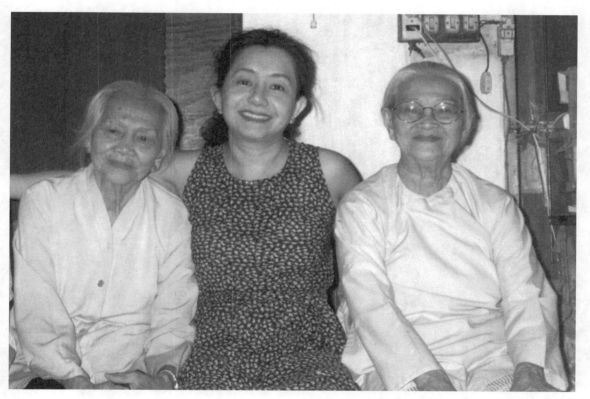

I visited my two aunts whom I call Ma Ba and Ma Nam (my two mothers). I was raised and spoiled by Ma Ba, who is 80, and Ma Nam, 78. Ma Nam has been a Buddhist vegetarian since she was 7 years old. Ma Ba on the other hand is just a part-time Buddhist vegetarian, which she only observes ten days a month. (Regular Buddhists believe that vegetarian food has a cleansing and calming effect on the body, and many choose to eat vegetarian food for two, four, or ten days of the lunar calendar.) I was taught very young to eat and love tofu and appreciate the benefit of it.

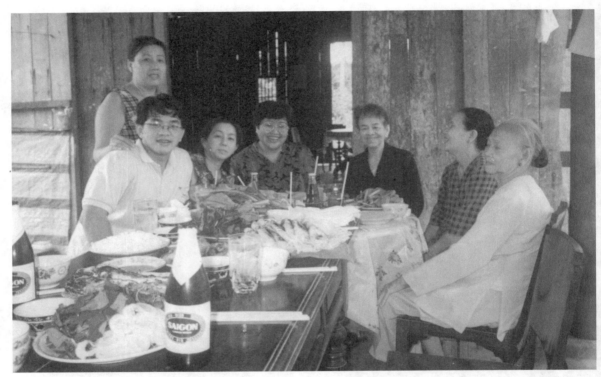

On my last Vietnam trip, I visited a co-worker 's family in Ben Tre, a province of South Vietnam. Her mother cooked us many traditional South Vietnamese dishes, which included abundant fresh vegetables, freshly caught fish, clams, and shrimp. It was the best lunch I have had in a long time.

The Asian Diet Menu Plan

If you want to start eating the Asian way, where do you start? The Asian daily pattern of eating is a bit different from the Western diet. At breakfast, Asians usually have a cup of coffee or tea and a bowl of fried, sweet, or black rice, a bowl of soup, or a piece of French bread. At lunch, we normally eat leftovers from the previous night's dinner or prepare something quick and easy. Snacks are optional and suited to individual preferences. Dinner is the main meal, and normally consists of rice, salad or a side vegetable, and one or two entrees, depending on the number of servings.

To help you plan your Asian diet, here are 18 days of suggested menus. Each day includes vegetarian (lacto-ovo) options. You'll notice that days 15 through 18 include a lighter lunch and heavier dinner. These menus were designed for weekends, since people tend to eat differently on the weekend from the way they eat on weekdays. Initially, dinners will take 30 to 45 minutes to prepare, but as you become more familiar with the cuisine, you will cut preparation time considerably. If your time is limited, you can double the recipe and package the leftovers for the next day's lunch or dinner, or you can freeze them for later use. My personal preference is to cook enough for dinner so that I have some left over for the next day's lunch.

Use these menus as a guide. You may want to follow days 1 through 6 from a Sunday to a Friday, and then day 15 for a Saturday. Or follow them in a different order, depending on how you eat during the week. If you prefer, mix and match recipes or choose other recipes listed at the end of the menus and contained in chapter 4. Just be sure that your total calories are between 1,200 and 1,400 (round down to 1,400 if total calories are 1,449 or less). Most women can lose weight on 1,200 to 1,400 calories, and we chose the 1,400-calorie level so you won't feel hungry and deprived and you'll lose weight safely. If you cut calories too much, you may lose weight more quickly, but such a plan usually backfires. Drastically cutting calories can lessen your chances of sticking with the program, so, although you may lose weight faster, you also run the risk of quickly regaining the weight you lost plus more.

Restricting calories too much also can cause a loss of lean (muscle) mass, which you don't want. Your metabolic rate is partly determined by the amount of lean mass you have. The more lean mass you lose, the lower your metabolic rate and the harder it becomes to maintain your weight. Note that the menus include many soups and vegetables. When trying to lose weight, adding soups and raw and cooked vegetables to meals is a good strategy. These foods are low in calories, packed with nutrients, and add bulk to the meal so you'll feel satisfied.

If you're going to restrict your calories by following these menus or a program of your own, make sure you take a multivitamin-mineral supplement. The supplement should provide up to 100 percent of nutritional requirements; there's no need to purchase a supplement that provides more than that. Vegetarians should make sure the supplement contains vitamin B12, because this vitamin is only found naturally in foods of animal origin.

The menus' calories have been calculated without adding sugar or cream to beverages. If you add sugar to any beverage, add 16 calories per teaspoon. If you add cream to any beverage, add 36 calories per tablespoon. We use 2 percent milk in the menus, but we recommend that, over time, you switch to 1 percent or skim milk. This will save you calories and fat. If you serve sauces with your meals (beyond what is listed on the menus), add the sauce calories to your total for the day.

How Fast Should You Lose?

You should lose about one to two pounds a week—the amount experts recommend as safe. We also advise you to follow the instructions below.

1. Don't eat fewer than 1,200 calories a day unless you are under the care of a physician and a registered dietitian.

2. Take a vitamin-mineral supplement that provides up to 100 percent of nutritional requirements. Vegetarians should ensure that the supplement contains vitamin B12, because this vitamin is only found naturally in foods of animal origin.

3. Remember that physical activity is a key ingredient of weight loss.

Day 1
Breakfast
3/4 cup unsweetened orange juice
(or other unsweetened juice)
1 ounce ready-to-eat cereal
1 cup 2% milk
coffee or tea
Calories: 301

Lunch
1 serving Asian Plain rice
1 serving Japanese Chicken Teriyaki
1 serving Korean/Japanese Ginger Pickles
water or tea
Calories: 450

Snack
1 apple
Calories: 80

Dinner
1 side dish serving Vietnamese Chicken Salad
1 serving Vietnamese Chicken Rice Soup with
Sweet and Sour Ginger Fish Sauce
1 slice Yucca Cake
Artichoke Tea
Calories: 597

Total Calories: 1,428

Day 1 Vegetarian Option
Breakfast
3/4 cup unsweetened orange juice (or other
unsweetened juice)
1 ounce ready-to-eat cereal
1 cup 2% milk
coffee or tea
Calories: 301

Lunch
1 serving Asian Brown Rice
1 serving Vietnamese Steamed Tofu with
Scallion Sauté

water or tea
Calories: 499

Snack
1 apple
Calories: 80

Dinner
1 serving Asian Plain Rice
1 serving Vegetable Ragout
1 slice Yucca Cake
Ginger Tea or Artichoke Tea
Calories 536

Total Calories: 1,416

Day 2
Breakfast
1 slice wheat bread, toasted
1 teaspoon jam
1 cup 2% milk
1 medium orange (or 1 piece any fresh fruit)
coffee or tea
Calories: 275

Lunch
1 main dish serving Vietnamese Chicken
Salad
1 medium orange (or 1 piece any fresh fruit)
tea or water
Calories: 401

Snack
1 cup coffee
Calories: 5

Dinner
1 serving Vietnamese Clear Vegetable Soup
(with shrimp)
1 serving Asian Plain Rice
1 serving Korean Barbecued Beef
1 serving Korean Kimchee
1 serving Korean Sesame Cucumber Salad

2 medium plums
tea or Artichoke Tea
Calories: 705

Total Calories: 1,386

Day 2 Vegetarian Option
Breakfast
1 slice wheat bread, toasted
1 teaspoon jam
1 cup 2% milk
1 medium orange (or 1 piece any fresh fruit)
coffee or tea
Calories: 275

Lunch
1 serving Vietnamese Vegetable Lomein
1/2 cup grapes
tea or water
Calories: 442

Snack
1 cup coffee
Calories: 5

Dinner
1 Vietnamese Vegetable Roll with
    Spicy Hoisin Sauce
1 serving Korean Cellophane Noodles with
    Vegetables
1 serving Vietnamese Banana and Yucca in
    Coconut Milk
tea or water
Calories: 602

Total Calories: 1,324

Day 3
Breakfast
1 serving Japanese Miso Soup
coffee or tea
Calories: 156

Lunch
3 Vietnamese Fresh Garden Rolls with
    Peanut Hoisin Sauce
1 grapefruit
tea or water
Calories: 500

Snack
1 cup hot or cold Soybean Milk
Calories: 193

Dinner
1 serving Chinese Chicken on Chicken-
    Flavored Rice with Sweet Ginger
    Soy Sauce
1 cup Chicken Broth
1 serving Chinese Cabbage Pickles
1 serving Korean Sesame Spinach
1/2 cup pineapple chunks (fresh or
    canned in juice)
tea or water
Calories: 528

Total Calories: 1,377

Day 3 Vegetarian Option
Breakfast
1 serving Japanese Miso Soup
coffee or tea
Calories: 156

Lunch
1 serving Vietnamese Tomato Rice
1 serving Mixed Vegetables
1 serving Vietnamese Fruit Shake (strawberry)
water
Calories: 489

Snack
1 cup hot or cold Soybean Milk
Calories: 193

Dinner

1 serving Vegetarian Pad Thai

1 serving Mixed Vegetables

1/2 cup melon

tea or water

Calories: 538

Total Calories: 1,376

Day 4
Breakfast

1/2 cup cooked cereal

1 cup 2% milk

12 medium strawberries (or 1 piece any fresh fruit)

coffee or tea

Calories: 242

Lunch

1 serving Chinese Chicken on Chicken-Flavored Rice with Sweet Ginger Soy Sauce

1 serving Korean Sesame Spinach

water or tea

Calories: 461

Snack

10 animal crackers

tea

Calories: 30

Dinner

1 serving Plain Rice

1 serving Chinese Fish Fillets in Sweet and Sour Lychee Sauce

1 serving Mixed Vegetables

1/2 cup fresh mango

tea or Artichoke Tea

Calories: 691

Total Calories: 1,424

Day 4 Vegetarian Option
Breakfast

1/2 cup cooked cereal

1 cup 2% milk

12 medium strawberries (or 1 piece any fresh fruit)

coffee or tea

Calories: 242

Lunch

1 serving Vegetarian Pad Thai

1 orange

tea

Calories: 441

Snack

10 animal crackers

tea

Calories: 58

Dinner

1 serving Asian Plain Rice

1 serving Indian Vegetarian Curry

1 serving Thai Mango Sticky Rice

2 kiwi fruit

tea

Calories: 628

Total Calories: 1,369

Day 5
Breakfast

1 serving Thai Mango Sticky Rice

coffee

Calories: 161

Lunch

1 serving Seafood Pad Thai Noodles

1 peach

tea

Calories: 432

Snack

1 serving Vietnamese Fruit Shake (orange)

Calories: 141

Dinner

1 serving Thai Squid Salad
1 serving Asian Plain Rice
1 serving Thai Pork in Spicy Basil Sauce
1 serving Mixed Vegetables
tea

Calories: 709

Total Calories: 1,443

Day 5 Vegetarian Option
Breakfast

1 serving Thai Mango Sticky Rice
coffee

Calories: 161

Lunch

1 serving Asian Plain Rice
1 serving Indian Vegetarian Curry
1 peach
tea or water

Calories: 414

Snack

1 serving Vietnamese Fruit Shake (orange)

Calories: 141

Dinner

1 serving Asian Plain Rice
1 serving Tofu Dip
1 serving Garden Salad
1 cup shredded Chinese cabbage, boiled
1 serving Vietnamese Vegetarian Hot and
    Sour Pineapple Soup
1 medium apple
tea

Calories: 564

Total Calories: 1,280

Day 6
Breakfast

1 frozen low-fat waffle
1 tablespoon apple butter
1/2 cup fresh orange and grapefruit sections
1 cup 2% milk
coffee

Calories: 278

Lunch

1 serving Asian Plain Rice
1 serving Thai Pork in Spicy Basil Sauce
1 serving Mixed Vegetables
tea

Calories: 575

Snack

1 plum
tea

Calories: 39

Dinner

1 side dish serving Vietnamese Mango Salad
1 serving Thai Flounder in Spicy Basil Sauce
1 serving Thai Hot and Sour Shrimp Soup
1 serving Garden Salad
tea

Calories: 541

Total Calories: 1,433

Day 6 Vegetarian Option
Breakfast

1 frozen low-fat waffle
1 tablespoon apple butter
1/2 cup fresh orange and grapefruit sections
1 cup 2% milk
coffee

Calories: 278

Lunch

1 serving Asian Plain Rice
1 serving Tofu Dip

1 serving Garden Salad
tea
Calories: 308

Snack
1 plum
tea
Calories: 39

Dinner
1 side dish serving Vietnamese Mango Salad
1 serving Vietnamese Vegetable Lomein
1 serving Chinese Black-Eyed Peas in Ginger
    and Orange-Flavored Syrup
1 tangerine
tea
Calories: 796

Total Calories: 1,421

Day 7
Breakfast
8 ounces nonfat light yogurt
1 tangerine
coffee
Calories: 162

Lunch
1 serving Asian Plain Rice
1 side dish serving Vietnamese Mango Salad
1 serving Thai Hot and Sour Shrimp Soup
tea
Calories: 412

Snack
1 cup hot or cold Soybean Milk
Calories: 193

Dinner
1 serving Asian Plain Rice
1 serving Vietnamese Salt and Pepper Shrimp
1 serving Vietnamese Asparagus in Tamarind
    Sauce

1 serving Vietnamese Clear Vegetable Soup
    with Pork
tea
Calories: 668

Total Calories: 1,435

Day 7 Vegetarian Option
Breakfast
8 ounces nonfat light yogurt
1 tangerine
coffee
Calories: 162

Lunch
1 side dish serving Vietnamese Mango Salad
1 serving Vietnamese Vegetable Lomein
tea or water
Calories: 534

Snack
1 cup hot or cold Soybean Milk
Calories: 193

Dinner
1 serving Korean Cellophane Noodles with
    Vegetables
1 serving Vietnamese Asparagus in Tamarind
    Sauce
Artichoke Tea
Calories: 510

Total Calories: 1,399

DAY 8
Breakfast
1 serving Vietnamese Fruit Shake (orange)
2 graham crackers (2-1/2-inch square)
Calories: 200

Lunch
1 serving Asian Plain Rice
1 serving Vietnamese Salt and Pepper Shrimp

1 serving Vietnamese Asparagus in Tamarind
Sauce
tea
Calories: 578

Snack
8 ounces vegetable juice cocktail
Calories: 46

Dinner
1 serving Asian Plain Rice
1 serving Vietnamese Five-Spice Pork Chops
1 serving Chinese Cabbage Pickles
1 serving Vietnamese Vegetarian Hot and
Sour Pineapple Soup
1/2 cup melon
tea
Calories: 576

Total Calories: 1,400

Day 8 Vegetarian Option
Breakfast
1 serving Vietnamese Fruit Shake (orange)
2 graham crackers (2-1/2-inch square)
Calories: 200

Lunch
1 serving Korean Cellophane Noodles with
Vegetables
1 serving Vietnamese Asparagus in Tamarind
Sauce
1 medium apple
tea or water
Calories: 586

Snack
8 ounces vegetable juice cocktail
Calories: 46

Dinner
1 serving Asian Plain Rice
1 serving Stir-Fried Vietnamese Garlic Chives

and Tofu
1 serving Thai Mango Sticky Rice
1/2 cup melon
tea
Calories: 558

Total Calories: 1,390

Day 9
Breakfast
1 serving Vietnamese Black Rice
1 medium orange
tea
Calories: 320

Lunch
1 serving Vietnamese Barbecued Lemongrass
Pork with Sweet and Sour Fish Sauce
1 serving Rice Vermicelli
tea
Calories: 443

Snack
4 ounces nonfat light fruit yogurt
Calories: 60

Dinner
1 serving Asian Plain Rice
1 side dish serving Vietnamese Papaya
Shrimp Salad
1 serving Chinese/Vietnamese Steamed Fish
in Hoisin Sauce
1 serving Thai Hot and Sour Shrimp Soup
1/2 cup grapes
tea
Calories: 617

Total Calories: 1,440

Day 9 Vegetarian Option
Breakfast
1 serving Vietnamese Black Rice
1 medium orange

tea
Calories: 320

Lunch
1 serving Asian Plain Rice
1 serving Stir-Fried Vietnamese Garlic Chives
and Tofu
tea
Calories: 371

Snack
4 ounces nonfat light fruit yogurt
Calories: 60

Dinner
1 serving Asian Plain Rice
1 serving Vietnamese Asparagus in Tamarind
Sauce
1 serving Vietnamese Spicy Lemongrass Tofu
1 serving Thai Hot and Sour Shrimp Soup
1/2 cup pineapple chunks (fresh or in juice)
Calories: 637

Total Calories: 1,388

Day 10
Breakfast
1/2 serving Vietnamese Chicken Noodle Soup
tea
Calories: 163

Lunch
1 main dish serving Vietnamese Papaya
Shrimp Salad
1 serving Vietnamese Vegetarian Hot and
Sour Pineapple Soup
water
Calories: 371

Snack
10 baby carrots
Calories: 38

Dinner
1 serving Japanese Miso Soup
1 serving Asian Plain Rice
1 serving Japanese Chicken Teriyaki
1 serving Korean/Japanese Ginger Pickles
1 serving Korean Sesame Cucumber Salad
1/2 cup mandarin orange sections
tea
Calories: 731

Total Calories: 1,303

Day 10 Vegetarian Option
Breakfast
1 serving Japanese Miso Soup
tea
Calories: 153

Lunch
1 serving Vietnamese Spicy Lemongrass Tofu
with Sweet and Sour Soy Sauce
1 serving Rice Vermicelli
tea
Calories: 348

Snack
10 baby carrots
Calories: 38

Dinner
1 serving Japanese Miso Soup
1 serving Asian Plain Rice
1 serving Thai Tofu and Green Beans in
Spicy Basil Sauce
1 serving Mixed Vegetables
1 slice Yucca Cake
1/2 cup blackberries
tea
Calories: 902

Total Calories: 1,441

Day 11

Breakfast

1 serving Vietnamese Fruit Shake (strawberry)

2 graham crackers (2-1/2-inch square)

tea

Calories: 187

Lunch

1 serving Vietnamese Pan-Fried Lemongrass Beef

1 serving Asian Plain Rice

1 medium apple

tea

Calories: 503

Snack

1 orange

1/2 cup grapes

Calories: 118

Dinner

1 serving Asian Plain Rice

1 serving Indian Chicken Curry

1/2 cup raspberries

tea

Calories: 482

Total Calories: 1,290

Day 11 Vegetarian Option

Breakfast

1 serving Vietnamese Fruit Shake (strawberry)

2 graham crackers (2-1/2-inch square)

tea

Calories: 187

Lunch

1 serving Asian Brown Rice

1 serving Thai Tofu and Green Beans in Spicy Basil Sauce

tea

Calories: 382

Snack

1 orange

1/2 cup grapes

Calories: 118

Dinner

1 serving Asian Plain Rice

1 serving Indian Vegetarian Curry

1 serving Chinese Soft Tofu in Ginger Sauce

tea

Calories: 706

Total Calories: 1,393

Day 12

Breakfast

1/2 cup cooked cereal

1 cup 2% milk

12 medium strawberries (or 1 piece any fresh fruit)

coffee or tea

Calories: 242

Lunch

1 serving Asian Plain Rice

1 serving Indian Chicken Curry

tea

Calories: 456

Snack

dried apricot halves

Artichoke Tea

Calories: 40

Dinner

1 serving Vietnamese Clear Vegetable Soup with Shrimp

1 serving Asian Plain Rice

1 serving Vietnamese Beef and Bean Sprouts

1 serving Vietnamese Ginger and Pineapple Salad

Artichoke Tea
Calories: 703

Total Calories: 1441

Day 12 Vegetarian Option
Breakfast
1/2 cup cooked cereal
1 cup 2% milk
12 medium strawberries (or 1 piece any fresh
   fruit)
coffee
Calories: 242

Lunch
1 serving Asian Plain Rice
1 serving Indian Vegetarian Curry
tea
Calories: 372

Snack
6 dried apricot halves
Artichoke Tea
Calories: 56

Dinner
1 serving Asian Plain Rice
1 serving Thai Tofu and Green Beans in
   Spicy Basil Sauce
1 serving Vietnamese Salt and Pepper
   Eggplant with Scallion Sauté
1 serving Thai Mango Sticky Rice
Artichoke Tea
Calories: 664

Total Calories: 1,334

Day 13
Breakfast
1 serving Thai Mango Sticky Rice
coffee
Calories: 161

Lunch
1 serving Asian Plain Rice
1 serving Thai Basil Beef and Broccoli
1 medium orange
tea
Calories: 689

Snack
1 cup cherry tomatoes
Calories: 31

Dinner
1 serving Asian Plain Rice
1 serving Vietnamese Pineapple Caramel
   Pork
1 serving Garden Salad
tea
Calories: 549

Total Calories: 1,430

Day 13 Vegetarian Option
Breakfast
1 serving Thai Mango Sticky Rice
coffee
Calories: 161

Lunch
1 serving Asian Plain Rice
1 serving Thai Tofu and Green Beans in
   Spicy Basil Sauce
tea
Calories: 380

Snack
1 cup cherry tomatoes
Calories: 31

Dinner
1 serving Japanese Miso Soup
1 serving Korean Cellophane Noodles with
   Vegetables
1 serving Korean Sesame Watercress

1 serving Chinese Black-Eyed Peas in Ginger
   and Orange-Flavored Syrup
tea
Calories: 738

Total Calories: 1,310

Day 14
Breakfast
8 ounces nonfat light fruit yogurt
1 fruit and cereal bar
1 tangerine (or 1 piece any fresh fruit)
coffee
Calories: 302

Lunch
1 serving Asian Plain Rice
1 serving Vietnamese Pineapple Caramel Pork
1 serving Korean Sesame Watercress
1/2 cup grapes
tea
Calories: 510

Snack
10 baby carrots
Calories: 38

Dinner
1 serving (appetizer portion) Thai Beef Satay
1 serving Thai Spicy Cucumber Salad
1 serving Vietnamese Bean Thread Noodles
   and Crabmeat
1 plum
tea
Calories: 589

Total Calories: 1,439

Day 14 Vegetarian Option
Breakfast
8 ounces nonfat light fruit yogurt
1 fruit and cereal bar

1 tangerine (or 1 piece any fresh fruit)
coffee
Calories: 302

Lunch
1 serving Korean Cellophane Noodles
   with Vegetables
1 serving Korean Sesame Watercress
1 medium banana
Calories: 471

Snack
10 baby carrots
Calories: 38

Dinner
3 Vietnamese Vegetable Rolls with
   Spicy Hoisin Sauce
1 serving Vietnamese Spicy Lemongrass Tofu
1 plum
tea
Calories: 461

Total Calories: 1,272

Day 15
Breakfast
1 serving Thai Coconut Sticky Rice
tea
Calories: 274

Lunch
2 Vietnamese Fresh Garden Rolls with
   Peanut Hoisin Sauce
2 kiwi fruit
tea
Calories: 378

Snack
1 glass Thai Iced Tea made with 2% milk
Calories: 146

Dinner

- 1 side dish serving Vietnamese Mango Salad
- 1 serving Vietnamese Catfish on Dill
- 1 serving Garden Salad
- 1 serving Vietnamese Banana and Yucca in Coconut Milk
- Artichoke Tea

Calories: 603

Total Calories: 1,401

Day 15 Vegetarian Option

Breakfast

- 1 serving Thai Coconut Sticky Rice
- tea

Calories: 274

Lunch

- 1 Vietnamese Vegetable Roll with Spicy Hoisin Sauce
- 1 medium pear
- tea

Calories: 203

Snack

- 1 glass Thai Iced Tea made with 2% milk

Calories: 146

Dinner

- 1 Vietnamese Vegetable Roll with Spicy Hoisin Sauce
- 1 serving Asian Plain Rice
- 1 serving Vegetable Ragout
- 1 serving Vietnamese Banana and Yucca in Coconut Milk
- Artichoke Tea

Calories: 627

Total Calories: 1,250

Day 16

Breakfast

- 1 egg, cooked without fat
- 1 slice wheat bread, toasted
- 1 teaspoon jam
- 1/2 cup cantaloupe (or 1 piece any fresh fruit)
- 1 cup 2% milk
- coffee or tea

Calories: 322

Lunch

- 1 serving Vietnamese Bean Thread Noodles and Crabmeat
- tea

Calories: 376

Snack

- 6 ounces tomato juice

Calories: 31

Dinner

- 1 Vietnamese Mung Bean and Shrimp Rice Cake
- 1 serving Vietnamese Beef Noodle Soup
- 1/2 cup pineapple chunks
- tea

Calories: 663

Total Calories: 1,392

Day 16 Vegetarian Option

Breakfast

- 1 egg, cooked without fat
- 1 slice wheat bread, toasted
- 1 teaspoon jam
- 1/2 cup cantaloupe (or 1 piece other fresh fruit)
- 1 cup 2% milk
- coffee or tea

Calories: 322

Lunch
1 serving Garlic Chives and Tofu Soup
1 serving Asian Brown Rice
1 serving Korean Sesame Spinach
tea
Calories: 420

Snack
6 ounces tomato juice
Calories: 31

Dinner
1 Chinese Mung Bean Rice Cake
1 serving Asian Plain Rice
1 serving Vegetable Ragout
1 slice Yucca Cake
tea
Calories: 667

Total Calories: 1,440

Day 17
Breakfast
1 serving Vietnamese Chicken Noodle Soup
coffee
Calories: 326

Lunch
1 serving Vietnamese Ginger and
    Pineapple Salad
tea
Calories: 89

Snack
1 serving Vietnamese Fruit Shake (strawberry)
Calories: 126

Dinner
1 serving Asian Plain Rice
1 serving Vietnamese Caramel Catfish in
    Clay Pot
1 serving Chinese Cabbage Pickles
1 serving Vietnamese Shrimp Pineapple Soup

1 medium apple
tea
Calories: 733

Total Calories: 1,274

Day 17 Vegetarian Option
Breakfast
1 serving Vietnamese Black Rice
coffee
Calories: 261

Lunch
1 serving Vietnamese Ginger and Pineapple
    Salad
tea
Calories: 89

Snack
1 serving Vietnamese Fruit Shake (strawberry)
Calories: 126

Dinner
1 serving Plain Fried Tofu
1 serving Asian Brown Rice
1 serving Vietnamese Salt and Pepper
    Eggplant with Scallion Sauté
1 serving Thai Tofu and Green Beans in
    Spicy Basil Sauce
1 serving Vietnamese Hot and Sour
    Pineapple Soup
1 orange
tea
Calories: 867

Total Calories: 1,343

Day 18
Breakfast
8 ounces nonfat light fruit yogurt
1 tangerine
coffee
Calories: 162

Lunch

1 serving Vietnamese Barbecued
Lemongrass Pork on Rice
1/2 cup mandarin orange sections
tea
Calories: 481

Snack

1 Asian pear
Calories: 51

Dinner

1 serving Asian Plain Rice
1 serving Chinese Chicken with
Mustard Greens
1 serving Vietnamese Pan-Fried
Lemongrass Beef
1 medium banana
tea
Calories: 755

Total Calories: 1,449

Nutrition analysis was completed using Food Processor software from ESHA Research, Inc.

Day 18 Vegetarian Option
Breakfast

8 ounces nonfat light fruit yogurt
1 tangerine
coffee
Calories: 162

Lunch

1 serving Vietnamese Spicy Lemongrass Tofu
1 serving Asian Brown Rice
tea
Calories: 346

Snack

1 Asian pear
Calories: 51

Dinner

1 serving Asian Plain Rice
1 serving Garden Salad
1 serving Thai Tofu and Green Beans in
Spicy Basil Sauce
1 serving Chinese Soft Tofu in Ginger Sauce
1/2 cup mandarin orange sections
tea
Calories: 815

Total Calories: 1,374

Recipe List
with Calorie Counts

Rice

Asian Plain Rice (277 calories)

Vietnamese Tomato Rice (236 calories)

Vietnamese Lemon Rice (244 calories)

Thai Coconut Sticky Rice (272 calories)

Vietnamese Black Rice (172 calories; 256 calories
with garnish)

Asian Brown Rice (228 calories)

Chinese Chicken-Flavored Rice (215 calories)

Appetizers

Vietnamese Fresh Garden Rolls with Peanut
Hoisin Sauce (141 calories)

Vietnamese Beef Rolls with Sweet and Sour
Fish Sauce (134 calories)

Vietnamese Mung Bean and Shrimp Rice
Cakes (155 calories)

Chinese Mung Bean Rice Cakes (136 calories)

Salads

Vietnamese Mango Salad (main dish:
244 calories; side dish: 122 calories)

Chinese Cabbage Pickles (22 calories)

Korean Kimchee (11 calories)

Thai Squid Salad (134 calories)

Vietnamese Asparagus Salad with Vinegar
Salad Dressing (115 calories)

Vietnamese Papaya Shrimp Salad (main dish:
211 calories; side dish: 106 calories)

Vietnamese Ginger and Pineapple Salad
(87 calories)

Korean/Japanese Ginger Pickles (7 calories)

Vietnamese Chicken Salad (main dish:
337 calories; side dish: 169 calories)

Korean Sesame Cucumber Salad (87 calories)

Thai Spicy Cucumber Salad (37 calories)

Garden Salad (57 calories)

Carrot Pickles (15 calories)

Soups

Vietnamese Chicken Noodle Soup (321 calories)

Vietnamese Beef Noodle Soup (468 calories)

Vietnamese Chicken or Duck Rice Soup with
Sweet and Sour Ginger Fish Sauce
(chicken: 216 calories; duck: 187 calories)

Thai Coconut Chicken Soup (108 calories)

Thai Hot and Sour Shrimp Soup (61 calories)

Vietnamese Chicken or Shrimp Pineapple
Soup (chicken: 131 calories; shrimp: 85 calories)

Japanese Miso Soup (150 calories)

Vietnamese Clear Vegetable Soup (shrimp:
29 calories; pork: 91 calories; beef: 82 calories;
turkey: 58 calories)

Beef Broth (14 calories)

Chicken Broth (14 calories)

Vegetable Broth (36 calories)

Main Dishes
Poultry

Chinese Chicken on Chicken-Flavored Rice
with Sweet Ginger Soy Sauce (374 calories)

Thai Chicken Satay (main dish: 164 calories;
appetizer or side dish: 82 calories)

Japanese Chicken Teriyaki (213 calories)

Vietnamese Ginger Chicken (180 calories)

Chinese Chicken with Mustard Greens
(228 calories)

Indian Chicken Curry (227 calories)

Vietnamese Chicken Ragout (158 calories)

Pork/Beef

Vietnamese Pineapple Caramel Pork
(167 calories)

Thai Pork in Spicy Basil Sauce (146 calories)

Vietnamese Five-Spice Pork Chops
(137 calories)

Vietnamese Pan-Fried Lemongrass Pork or
Beef (pork: 142 calories; beef: 189 calories)

Vietnamese Barbecued Lemongrass Pork or Beef on Rice Vermicelli (pork: 415 calories; beef: 484 calories)

Korean Barbecued Beef (272 calories)

Thai Beef Satay (appetizer: 197 calories; main dish: 334 calories)

Korean Beef (281 calories)

Vietnamese Beef and Bean Sprouts (354 calories)

Thai Basil Beef and Broccoli (398 calories)

Seafood

Vietnamese Bean Thread Noodles and Crabmeat (main dish: 376 calories; side dish: 188 calories)

Chinese Fish Fillets in Sweet and Sour Lychee Sauce (276 calories)

Chinese/Vietnamese Steamed Fish in Hoisin Sauce (165 calories)

Vietnamese Salt and Pepper Shrimp (148 calories)

Vietnamese Catfish on Dill (221 calories)

Thai Flounder in Spicy Basil Sauce (298 calories)

Vietnamese Caramel Catfish in Clay Pot (317 calories)

Seafood Pad Thai Noodles (358 calories)

Vegetables/Vegetarian Delights

Plain Fried Tofu (141 calories)

Vietnamese Steamed Tofu with Scallion Sauté (269 calories)

Indian Vegetarian Curry (143 calories)

Vietnamese Spicy Lemongrass Tofu (116 calories)

Korean Cellophane Noodles with Vegetables (232 calories)

Korean Sesame Spinach (83 calories) or Watercress (58 calories)

Vietnamese Salt and Pepper Eggplant with Scallion Sauté (123 calories)

Thai Eggplant in Spicy Basil Sauce (110 calories)

Vegetarian Pad Thai (377 calories)

Vietnamese Asparagus in Tamarind Sauce (201 calories)

Vietnamese Vegetarian Hot and Sour Pineapple Soup (159 calories)

Vegetable Ragout (97 calories)

Vietnamese Vegetable Lomein (410 calories)

Thai Tofu and Green Beans in Spicy Basil Sauce (151 calories)

Stir-Fried Vietnamese Garlic Chives and Tofu (141 calories)

Garlic Chives and Tofu Soup (107 calories)

Tofu Dip (22 calories)

Vietnamese Vegetable Rolls with Spicy Hoisin Sauce (93 calories)

Mixed Vegetables (128 calories)

Desserts

Thai Mango Sticky Rice (156 calories)

Chinese Black-Eyed Peas in Ginger and Orange-Flavored Syrup (225 calories)

Chinese Soft Tofu in Ginger Sauce (335 calories)

Vietnamese Banana and Yucca in Coconut Milk (195 calories)

Yucca Cake (206 calories)

Beverages

Vietnamese Fruit Shake (strawberry: 126 calories; orange: 141 calories; pineapple: 141 calories)

Thai Iced Tea (with half-and-half or evaporated milk: 171 calories; with 2% milk: 146 calories)

Artichoke Tea (with sugar: 23 calories; without sugar: 6 calories)

Ginger Tea (4 calories)

Soybean Milk (with sugar: 210 calories; without sugar: 193 calories)

PART 2

Eating the Asian Way

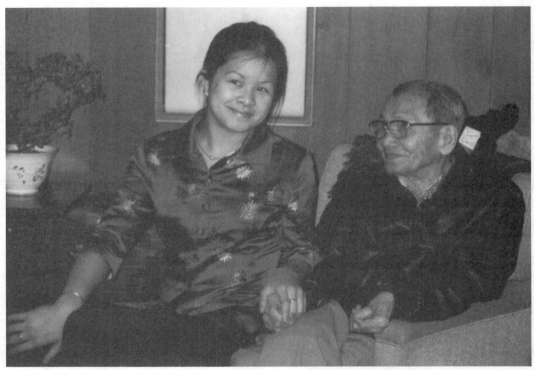

Cooking for my family, with the three genera-
tions, is a challenge. I am fortunate that my
father is becoming more westernized and my
daughter still values Vietnamese traditions. I
am able to use some old recipes as well as
some adapted western recipes to please both.

4 Favorite Asian Recipes

CHAPTER 4

Getting Started

Equipment

Asian cooking requires some special, readily available equipment. You will need a wok or nonstick stir-fry pan, steamer, food processor, mixer, two soup pots, nonstick saucepans, and, if possible, an electric rice cooker. Sharp knives and/or a cleaver for cutting and chopping are essential.

Ingredients

Asian cuisine is becoming very popular in America. Many essential ingredients, such as fish sauce, oyster sauce, soy sauce, hoisin sauce, soybean paste, teriyaki sauce, all types of Asian rice, noodles, mushrooms, and traditional spices and herbs, are available in the foreign/ethnic food section of your local supermarket and in Asian markets.

Tips

Cooking Asian foods may be a challenge at first, but it will become much easier and faster as you gain experience. I include some of my favorite Asian recipes and the tips that help perfect them.

Rice is the main part of an Asian meal. Making perfect rice is important, and it can be cooked easily with an electric rice cooker available in any Asian or department store. When you buy rice in an Asian store, ask whether it is newly harvested because, if it is, it takes less water than the rice that is not fresh. If you buy it in a local supermarket, use the long-grain variety and experiment to find the correct amount of water needed. The rice should be moist, not wet or dry, and fluffy.

Sweet rice (also called sticky rice) needs to be soaked overnight if you use a steamer.

A variety of sauces accompany every meal. The best known is fish sauce. Southeast Asians use plain fish sauce for cooking and sometimes for table sauce. It is salty and could be substituted with salt. Sweet and sour fish sauce is paired primarily with Vietnamese and/or

Thai entrées. Add more or less sugar, lime, water, or pepper to your individual taste. Chinese, Japanese, and Koreans prefer soy sauce or soybean paste. Teriyaki sauce is used more in Korean and Japanese cooking. Chinese cuisine favors soy, black bean, and oyster sauces. Chinese dishes normally are accompanied by a bowl of red vinegar and soy sauce. I recommend that red vinegar be served with meat or seafood dishes.

Rice

Asian Plain Rice
(3 servings)

1 cup long-grain jasmine rice
1-1/4 cups water

1. Wash rice until water runs clear, then drain.

2. In small nonstick saucepan, add rice and water. Bring to a boil, turn down heat to medium, and cook until all water is absorbed, about seven minutes, stirring gently once or twice. Cover tightly, turn heat to very low, and cook until tender, about 15 to 20 minutes.

3. Before serving, fluff rice with chopsticks or a fork.

To serve: Asians serve rice with any main course, in small individual bowls with chopsticks.

Nutrition Information per Serving: 277 calories, 0 g total fat (0 g saturated fat), 0 mg cholesterol, 3 mg sodium, 51 g carbohydrates, 1 g dietary fiber, 4 g protein

Vietnamese Tomato Rice

(3 servings)

1 cup long-grain jasmine rice
1-1/4 cups water
1/4 teaspoon salt
1/4 teaspoon garlic powder or 1 garlic clove finely minced
1/2 teaspoon olive oil
1 tablespoon tomato sauce

1. Wash rice until water runs clear, then drain.

2. Mix rice, water, salt, garlic, oil, and tomato sauce in a nonstick saucepan and bring to a boil. Turn heat down to very low, stir gently, cover tightly, and cook until tender, about 15 to 20 minutes.

3. Before serving, stir rice with chopsticks or a fork to be sure it is evenly moist.

To serve: Serve steaming hot with any seafood, meat, or chicken dish.

Nutrition Information per Serving: 236 calories, 1 g total fat (0.1 g saturated fat), 0 mg cholesterol, 228 mg sodium, 51 g carbohydrates, 1 g dietary fiber, 4 g protein

Vietnamese Lemon Rice

(3 servings)

1 cup long-grain jasmine rice
1-1/4 cups water
1/4 teaspoon salt
1 teaspoon olive oil
zest of half a lemon
1/2 teaspoon lemon juice

1. Wash rice until water runs clear, then drain.

2. Mix rice, water, salt, and oil in a nonstick saucepan and bring to a boil. Turn heat down to very low, stir gently, cover tightly, and cook until tender, about 15 to 20 minutes.

3. Add lemon zest and juice and mix lightly with chopsticks or a fork.

To serve: Serve steaming hot with any seafood, meat, or chicken dish.

Nutrition Information per Serving: 244 calories, 2 g total fat (0.2 g saturated fat), 0 mg cholesterol, 197 mg sodium, 52 g carbohydrates, 2 g dietary fiber, 4 g protein

Thai Coconut Sticky Rice
(3 servings)

1 cup glutinous rice
1/2 cup water
1/2 cup coconut milk
1/4 teaspoon salt
1 tablespoon oil

1. In a nonstick saucepan, combine rice, water, coconut milk, salt, and oil and bring to a boil. Turn heat down immediately and stir gently. Cover tightly, turn down heat to very low, and cook until done, about 20 minutes. Before serving, stir rice to be sure it is evenly moist.

2. If using a steamer, omit water. Toss rice, coconut milk, salt, and oil in a steamer. Steam 20 minutes.

To serve: Serve by itself or with entrées. Add sugar if preferred. Serve as a dessert with mangoes and Coconut Sauce (see Thai Mango Sticky Rice, p. 137).

Nutrition Information per Serving: 272 calories, 5 g total fat (1 g saturated fat), 0 mg cholesterol, 218 mg sodium, 51 g carbohydrates, 2 g dietary fiber, 4 g protein

Vietnamese Black Rice
(2 servings)

1/2 cup black rice
1 cup water

Garnish (optional):
1/2 cup shredded coconut
1/2 tablespoon sesame seeds

1. Soak black rice in warm water for at least four hours, preferably overnight, then drain.

2. Combine black rice and water in a nonstick saucepan. Bring to a boil. Turn heat to medium and simmer until all water is absorbed, about 40 minutes. If you prefer to use a rice steamer, the rice must be soaked overnight. Place rice in a steamer over boiling water and steam 40 minutes until tender.

To serve: Enjoy Black Rice with baked meats or poultry for dinner. To serve as breakfast or a sweet snack, sprinkle with shredded coconut, toasted sesame seeds, and a little sugar to taste.

Nutrition Information per Serving of Black Rice: 172 calories, 1 g total fat (0 g saturated fat), 0 mg cholesterol, 5 mg sodium, 36 g carbohydrates, 0 g dietary fiber, 4 g protein

Nutrition Information per Serving of Garnish: 84 calories, 8 g total fat (6 g saturated fat), 0 mg cholesterol, 4 mg sodium, 4 g carbohydrates, 2 g dietary fiber, 1 g protein

Asian Brown Rice
(3 servings)

1 cup brown rice
3 cups spring water

1. Wash brown rice until the water runs clear, then drain.

2. In a nonstick saucepan, add brown rice and spring water. Bring to a boil, turn down heat to medium, and cook until all water is absorbed, stirring gently once or twice. Cover tightly, turn heat to very low and cook until tender, about 40 minutes more.

3. Before serving, fluff rice with chopstick or a fork.

To serve: Serve brown rice with any entrée in place of white rice or by itself with crushed sesame seeds.

Nutrition Information per Serving: 228 calories, 2 g total fat (0.4 g saturated fat), 0 mg cholesterol, 7 mg sodium, 48 g carbohydrates, 2 g dietary fiber, 5 g protein

Chinese Chicken-Flavored Rice

(4 servings)

1-1/4 cups long-grain jasmine rice

1-1/4 cups chicken broth

1 2-inch cinnamon stick (optional)

1. Wash rice until the water runs clear, then drain.

2. In a small nonstick saucepan, add rice, chicken broth, and cinnamon stick (if preferred). Bring to a boil, turn down heat to medium, and cook until all water is absorbed, about seven minutes, stirring gently once or twice. Cover tightly, turn heat to very low, and cook until tender, about 15 to 20 minutes more.

3. Before serving, fluff rice with chopsticks or a fork.

To serve: Serve with Chinese Chicken (p. 82) or any other entrée.

Nutrition Information per Serving: 215 calories, 0 g total fat (0 g saturated fat), 0 mg cholesterol, 37 mg sodium, 48 g carbohydrates, 1 g dietary fiber, 4 g protein

Appetizers

Vietnamese Fresh Garden Rolls with Peanut Hoisin Sauce

(8 rolls, 1 roll per serving)

2 ounces dry rice vermicelli (yields about 1/2 cup cooked)

1/4 pound lean, boneless pork

1 cup water

15 medium-size shrimp

5 leaves lettuce (such as romaine)

5 sprigs garlic chives (available in Asian grocery stores)

1 cup bean sprouts

5 mint sprigs

5 basil sprigs

5 cilantro sprigs

8 8-inch round rice papers

Peanut Hoisin Sauce (see below)

1. Bring a large saucepan of water to a boil. Add rice vermicelli and, stirring gently, cook until the noodles are transparent and soft, about five minutes. Drain and rinse under cold running water. Drain again thoroughly and set aside.

2. Cut the pork into 1-inch-thick strips. In a medium saucepan, simmer pork strips in one cup water for about 15 minutes, until they are well done. Remove pork strips and reserve stock. When cool, cut strips into narrow slices. Using the same saucepan, heat reserved stock, add shrimp, and cook about three minutes, until they are pink and curled. Remove shrimp, cool, devein, and set aside. Reserve stock for use in Peanut Hoisin Sauce.

3. Wash lettuce leaves and tear them in half. Wash garlic chives and cut each into two long strips. Wash bean sprouts and drain thoroughly. Strip leaves from mint, basil, and cilantro sprigs; wash and pat dry.

4. On your work surface, assemble all ingredients, as well as a pastry brush, a bowl of warm water, and a dampened dish towel or paper towel. Using pastry brush dipped in warm water, dampen the entire surface of three pieces of rice paper, putting each one on the damp towel. Working with three pieces at a time, place the following in a 6-inch row one inch from the edge nearest you: half a romaine lettuce leaf, a few herbs, a little vermicelli, and three pieces each of meat and shrimp. Fold the left and right sides of the rice paper inward. Insert two garlic chive strips about 7 inches long. Fold the bottom, nearest edge over the filling, while pressing down on the mixture, and roll as tightly as possible to top edge. Repeat the procedure with the remaining ingredients. Cover rolls with plastic wrap so they don't dry out and set aside until serving time.

5. Prepare Peanut Hoisin Sauce.

To serve: Each person should be served an individual bowl of Peanut Hoisin Sauce (see below).

Nutrition Information per Roll (without Peanut Hoisin Sauce): 101 calories, 1 g total fat (0.4 g saturated fat), 26 mg cholesterol, 190 mg sodium, 15 g carbohydrates, 1 g dietary fiber, 7 g protein

Peanut Hoisin Sauce

Yield: 1 cup (2 tablespoons per serving)

1/2 cup shrimp and pork stock

1/4 cup milk

3 tablespoons hoisin sauce

1/2 tablespoon red chile sauce (optional)

1 tablespoon crunchy peanut butter

1/2 tablespoon sugar

1 teaspoon cornstarch

1 tablespoon crushed peanuts for garnish

1. In a saucepan, mix the stock, milk, hoisin sauce, red chile sauce, crunchy peanut butter, and sugar. Bring to a boil and immediately turn heat down to low.

2. In a small bowl, mix water and cornstarch. Pour into the saucepan and stir constantly until sauce is thick and creamy. Garnish with crushed peanuts before serving.

To serve: Serve with Vietnamese Fresh Garden Rolls. Sprinkle crushed peanuts and pass red chili sauce to taste.

Nutrition Information per Serving: 40 calories, 2 g total fat (0.4 g saturated fat), 1 mg cholesterol, 158 mg sodium, 5 g carbohydrates, 0 g dietary fiber, 1 g protein

Vietnamese Beef Rolls
with Sweet and Sour Fish Sauce

(8 rolls; 1 roll per serving)

1 teaspoon oil	4 mint sprigs
1 garlic clove, minced	4 basil sprigs
1/2 medium onion, chopped	4 cilantro sprigs
1/2 cup ground beef	1 cup bean sprouts
1/8 cup peanuts, crushed	1/2 cup cooked rice vermicelli
pinch of salt	8 8-inch round rice papers
1/4 teaspoon black pepper	Sweet and Sour Fish Sauce
pinch of sugar	(see below)
4 leaves romaine lettuce	Red cayenne pepper, thinly sliced

1. Over medium flame, heat oil in a fry pan. Brown garlic, then stir in chopped onion and cook until soft. Add ground beef, crushed peanuts, salt, pepper, and sugar and stir until meat is well done.

2. Proceed as for Vietnamese Fresh Garden Rolls (p. 43), beginning at instruction number 3.

3. Prepare Sweet and Sour Fish Sauce.

To serve: Dip Beef Rolls into individual bowl of Sweet and Sour Fish Sauce (below). Add more sliced red cayenne pepper to taste.

Nutrition Information per Roll (without Sweet and Sour Fish Sauce): 109 calories, 4 g total fat (1 g saturated fat), 10 mg cholesterol, 203 mg sodium, 13 g carbohydrates, 1 g dietary fiber, 5 g protein

Sweet and Sour Fish Sauce

Yield: 1 cup (2 tablespoons per serving)

2 garlic cloves, finely minced

3 tablespoons sugar

2 tablespoons lime or lemon juice

1/2 cup warm water

6 tablespoons fish sauce

1/2 teaspoon ground red chile pepper, or to taste

1. In a small bowl, mix the minced garlic, sugar, lime or lemon juice, water, and fish sauce until sugar has completely dissolved. Add ground red chile pepper as desired.

To serve: Serve with almost any entrée.

Nutrition Information per Serving: 25 calories, 0 g total fat (0 g saturated fat), 0 mg cholesterol, 1043 mg sodium, 6 g carbohydrates, 0 g dietary fiber, 1 g protein

Vietnamese Mung Bean and Shrimp Rice Cakes

(12 cakes; 1 cake per serving)

Filling:

1/2 cup dry mung beans

1/2 cup water

1 teaspoon oil

1 garlic clove, minced

1/2 cup onion, finely chopped

1/2 cup pork shoulder, cooked and
    thinly sliced

10 medium-size shrimp, shelled
    and chopped

1/4 teaspoon salt

1/4 teaspoon pepper

1/2 teaspoon sugar

1/2 teaspoon fish sauce

Scallion Sauté (see below)

1 teaspoon oil

2 scallions, finely sliced

Rice Cake Dough:

2 cups (1/2 pound) glutinous rice
    flour

1 cup warm water

1 tablespoon oil

aluminum foil, cut into 12 2-inch x
    2-inch squares

1. Soak dry mung beans in a saucepan of warm water. Set aside for
   one hour.

2. Rinse mung beans thoroughly in a colander and drain.

3. In a nonstick saucepan, mix mung beans and 1/2 cup water. Bring to
   a boil, uncovered, over medium-low heat, stirring gently. Cover
   saucepan tightly, turn heat to very low and cook until mung beans
   are dry and fluffy, approximately 15 minutes. Cool and set aside.

4. In a large frying pan, heat 1 teaspoon oil and brown garlic and onion.
   Add pork, shrimp, salt, pepper, and sugar and stir-fry for five minutes.
   Add cooked mung beans and fish sauce. Stirring constantly, mash
   beans with the back of a large spoon until all ingredients are well
   mixed. Cool and set aside for 10 minutes. Meanwhile, prepare dough.

5. In a large bowl, mix glutinous rice flour with water, knead until
   smooth. Divide dough into 12 equal portions.

6. Prepare your workstation. Lightly oil the 12 aluminum foil squares. Pour remaining oil into a small bowl.

7. Oil your hands and form the mung bean mixture into 12 balls, each 1-1/2 inches in diameter.

8. Use your palms to flatten each ball of rice flour dough into a 2-inch circle. Place a mung bean ball in the center of the circle of dough, then mold the dough around it to enclose the bean ball completely. With oiled palms, gently roll each ball clockwise until it is smooth and rounded. Place each ball on an oiled foil square. The oiled squares keep the cakes from sticking to the steamer.

9. Arrange 6 mung bean balls 1 inch apart in a steamer. Bring water to a boil, cover, and steam each batch for 10 minutes; set aside until cool enough to handle.

10. For Scallion Sauté, heat oil over medium heat and stir-fry scallions for 1 minute. Remove from heat and set aside until serving time.

To serve: Oil your hands first because the balls are very sticky, then remove foil and arrange the balls on a lightly oiled plate. The mung bean balls can be served alone, garnished with Scallion Sauté and/or with Sweet and Sour Fish Sauce (p. 47).

Nutrition Information per Cake with Scallion Sauté: 155 calories, 3 g total fat (1 g saturated fat), 9 mg cholesterol, 77 g sodium, 26 g carbohydrates, 2 g dietary fiber, 5 g protein

Scallion Sauté Nutriton information per serving: 4 calories, 0 g total fat (0 g saturated fat), 0 mg cholesterol, 0 g sodium, 0 g carbohydrate, 0 g dietary fiber, 0 g protein

Chinese Mung Bean Rice Cakes
(12 cakes; 1 cake per serving)

Filling:
1/2 cup dry mung beans
1/2 cup water
1 teaspoon oil
1 garlic clove, minced
1/2 cup onion, finely chopped
1/2 teaspoon salt
1/4 teaspoon pepper
1/2 teaspoon sugar

Rice Cake Dough:
2 cups (1/2 pound) glutinous rice flour
1 cup warm water
1 tablespoon oil
aluminum foil, cut into 12 2-inch x 2-inch squares

1. Soak dry mung beans in a saucepan of warm water. Set aside for one hour.

2. Rinse mung beans thoroughly in a colander and drain.

3. In a nonstick saucepan, mix mung beans and 1/2 cup water. Bring to a boil, uncovered, over medium-low heat, stirring gently. Cover saucepan tightly, turn heat to very low, and cook until mung beans are dry and fluffy, approximately 15 minutes. Cool and set aside.

4. In a large frying pan, heat 1 teaspoon oil and brown garlic and onion. Add salt, pepper, and sugar and stir-fry for 5 minutes. Add cooked mung beans. Stirring constantly, mash beans with the back of a large spoon until all ingredients are well mixed. Cool and set aside for 10 minutes. Meanwhile, prepare dough.

5. In a large bowl, mix glutinous rice flour with warm water, knead until smooth. Divide dough into 12 equal portions.

6. Prepare your workstation. Lightly oil the 12 aluminum foil squares. Pour remaining oil into a small bowl.

7. Oil your hands and form the mung bean mixture into 12 balls.

8. Use your palms to flatten each ball of rice flour dough into a 2-inch circle. Place a mung bean ball in the center of the circle of dough, molding dough around it to enclose the bean ball completely. With oiled palms, gently roll each ball clockwise until it is smooth and rounded. Place each ball on an oiled foil square. The oiled squares keep the cakes from sticking to the steamer.

9. Arrange 6 mung bean balls 1 inch apart in a steamer. Bring water to a boil, cover, and steam each batch for 10 minutes; set aside until cool enough to handle.

To serve: Oil your hands first because the balls are very sticky, then remove foil and arrange the balls on a lightly oiled plate. The mung bean balls can be served alone or with Sweet and Sour Fish Sauce (p. 47) or Sweet and Sour Soy Sauce (p. 136).

Nutrition Information per Cake: 136 calories, 2 g total fat (0.4 g saturated fat), 0 mg cholesterol, 98 mg sodium, 26 g carbohydrates, 2 g dietary fiber, 3 g protein

Salads

Vietnamese Mango Salad
(2 main dish servings; 4 side dish servings)

2 green mangoes, sliced lengthwise and coarsely shredded
   (yields about 4 cups)
10 shrimp
1/4 teaspoon salt
1 tablespoon sugar
1 tablespoon fish sauce
1 red chile pepper, thinly sliced (optional)
2 tablespoons Sweet and Sour Fish Sauce (p. 47)
shrimp paste chips or tortilla chips

Garnish:
5 mint sprigs or Cayang sprigs, minced
1 tablespoon crushed peanuts

1. In a small saucepan, add water to cover shrimp and cook about 5 minutes. Drain shrimp and devein when cool enough. Set aside.

2. In a large bowl, toss together the shredded mangoes, salt, sugar, fish sauce, and chile pepper. Refrigerate until serving time.

3. Remove salad mixture from refrigerator, add two tablespoons of Sweet and Sour Fish Sauce (p. 47), and toss again.

To serve: Garnish with shrimp, mint, and peanuts. Serve by itself or with shrimp paste chips or tortilla chips, Sweet and Sour Fish Sauce, and more thinly sliced red chile pepper.

Nutrition Information per Serving (as a main dish): 244 calories, 3 g total fat (1 g saturated fat), 46 mg cholesterol, 1581 mg sodium, 46 g carbohydrates, 5 g dietary fiber, 10 g protein

Nutrition Information per Serving (as a side dish): 122 calories, 2 g total fat (.6 g saturated fat), 23 mg cholesterol, 790 mg sodium, 23 g carbohydrates, 2 g dietary fiber, 5 g protein

Chinese Cabbage Pickles
(15 servings)

1 medium head cabbage
1/2 cup salt
1 cup warm water
1/2 cup white vinegar
2 tablespoons sugar
2 garlic cloves, finely minced
2 inches ginger, finely minced

1. Cut the cabbage into pieces about 1-1/2 inches long by 1-1/2 inches wide.

2. In a large bowl, mix the salt with water to cover. Soak the cabbage in the salt water, tossing it occasionally to ensure all parts are well submerged. Set aside for 30 minutes.

3. In a small bowl, beat together 1 cup warm water, vinegar, and sugar until sugar is completely dissolved. Set aside.

4. Rinse and drain the cabbage. Transfer the cabbage to a large mixing bowl. Add minced garlic, minced ginger, and vinegar mixture and toss well. Reserve liquid from mixture.

5. Pack the marinated cabbage into large glass jars and pour the reserved liquid mixture into the jars. Cap the jars tightly and store them at room temperature about 24 hours, then in the refrigerator. Cabbage should be ready in 48 hours. Keep refrigerated so the cabbage won't take on a more sour flavor.

To serve: Serve as a side dish to accompany any entrée.

Nutrition Information per Serving: 22 calories, 0 g total fat (0 g saturated fat), 0 mg cholesterol, 477 mg sodium, 5 g carbohydrates, 1 g dietary fiber, 1 g protein

Korean Kimchee

(20 servings)

1 medium head Chinese cabbage

1/2 cup salt for soaking

1 cup warm water

2 cloves garlic, finely minced

2-inch piece ginger, peeled and finely minced

1 tablespoon red pepper powder

1 fresh hot red pepper, thinly sliced

2 scallions, cut into 2-inch strips

1 tablespoon sugar

1. Cut the cabbage into pieces about 1-1/2 inches long by 1-1/2 inches wide.

2. In a large bowl, mix the salt with water to cover. Soak the cabbage in the salt water, tossing it occasionally to ensure all parts are well submerged. Set aside for 4 hours.

3. Rinse and drain the cabbage. Transfer the cabbage into a large bowl. Combine 1 cup warm water, minced garlic, minced ginger, red pepper powder, fresh hot red pepper, scallion strips, and sugar and toss well. Reserve liquid from mixture.

4. Pack the marinated cabbage into large glass jars. Pour in the remaining liquid from the mixture. Keep jars tightly capped at room temperature for about 24 hours, then store them in the refrigerator. Kimchee should be ready in 48 hours. Keep kimchee refrigerated so it will not take on an even more sour flavor.

To serve: Serve as a side dish to accompany any entrée.

Nutrition Information per Serving: 11 calories, 0 g total fat (0 g saturated fat), 0 mg cholesterol, 377 mg sodium, 2 g carbohydrates, 1 g dietary fiber, 1 g protein

Thai Squid Salad
(4 servings)

1 pound fresh or frozen squid, cleaned (also called calamari)
4 garlic cloves, finely minced
2 red chile hot peppers, thinly sliced
1 small onion, thinly sliced
3 tablespoons lime juice
2 tablespoons fish sauce
1/2 teaspoon sugar
1/4 teaspoon salt
5 sprigs mint, finely chopped
5 sprigs cilantro, finely chopped
4 large lettuce leaves

1. Wash and clean fresh or frozen squid. Drain and cut into 1-inch rings. Bring 6 cups water to a boil in a medium saucepan. Add the squid to the boiling water and blanch about 1 minute, stirring occasionally. Do not overcook. Rinse under cold running water, drain, and set aside.

2. In a large mixing bowl, toss together cooked squid, garlic, red chile hot peppers, onion, lime juice, fish sauce, sugar, and salt. Set aside at least 20 minutes.

To serve: Before serving, toss all ingredients well. Transfer squid to a plate lined with lettuce leaves. Sprinkle mint, cilantro, and thinly sliced red hot chile pepper.

Nutrition Information per Serving: 134 calories, 2 g total fat (0.4 g saturated fat), 264 mg cholesterol, 896 mg sodium, 10 g carbohydrates, 1 g dietary fiber, 19 g protein

Vietnamese Asparagus Salad with Vinegar Salad Dressing

(2 servings)

10 stalks fresh asparagus
1/2 medium tomato
1/2 teaspoon olive oil
1 scallion, chopped
1 tablespoon roasted, unsalted sesame seeds
1/2 cup Vinegar Salad Dressing (see below)

1. Thoroughly wash and trim asparagus, and cut into 2-inch pieces. In a medium saucepan, bring water to a boil and cook asparagus for three minutes. In a colander, quickly rinse asparagus under cold running water and drain thoroughly.

2. Seed tomato and dice.

3. Heat olive oil over medium heat, add chopped scallions, and stir-fry for a few seconds. Remove scallions from heat and set aside.

4. Toss all ingredients with Vinegar Salad Dressing (below). Chill until serving time.

To serve: Toss just before serving to combine well and arrange on serving plates.

Nutrition Information per Serving: 96 calories, 4 g total fat (1 g saturated fat), 0 mg cholesterol, 305 mg sodium, 13 g carbohydrates, 3 g dietary fiber, 3 g protein

Vinegar Salad Dressing

Yield: 1 cup (16 tablespoons; 2 tablespoons per serving)

1/2 cup white or apple vinegar
1 teaspoon olive oil
1/4 cup water
1/2 teaspoon salt
1/2 teaspoon pepper
1-1/2 tablespoons sugar
2 garlic cloves, finely minced
1 small red or white onion, thinly sliced

1. In a medium bowl, beat together the vinegar, olive oil, water, salt, pepper, and sugar. When sugar is completely dissolved, pour over the garlic and thinly sliced onion and toss well.

To serve: Serve this dressing with any salads, Western or Asian.

Nutrition Information per Serving: 19 calories, 1 g total fat (0 g saturated fat), 0 mg cholesterol, 149 mg sodium, 3 g carbohydrates, 0 g dietary fiber, 0 g protein

Vietnamese Papaya Shrimp Salad
(2 main dish servings; 4 side dish servings)

1/8 pound boneless pork, cut into 1-inch-thick strips

10 shrimp

1/2 medium-size green papaya

1 carrot

1/2 teaspoon salt for soaking

1 red chile pepper, thinly sliced (optional)

5 cilantro sprigs, minced

5 mint sprigs, minced

1 tablespoon crushed peanuts

1/2 cup Vinegar Salad Dressing (p. 57)

3 tablespoons Sweet and Sour Fish Sauce (p. 47)

shrimp paste chips or tortilla chips

1. In a medium saucepan, simmer the pork strips in water to barely cover for about 20 minutes or until well done. Remove pork strips, reserving stock, and cool the strips before slicing them into thin pieces. Reheat the same saucepan for the shrimp and cook them about 5 minutes. Drain shrimp and devein when cool enough. Set aside.

2. Peel papaya and cut into two pieces. Finely shred papaya and carrot.

3. In a deep pan, cover papaya and carrot with cold water and salt. Set aside for 20 minutes, then rinse with cold water, drain, and dry.

4. Add the red chile pepper to the Vinegar Salad Dressing (p. 57).

5. Reserve some of the pork, shrimp, cilantro, mint, and peanuts for garnish. In a large bowl, toss together the shredded papaya, carrot, remaining pork, shrimp, herbs, and peanuts, add the salad dressing, and toss. Refrigerate until serving time.

6. Remove salad mixture from refrigerator, add 3 tablespoons Sweet and Sour Fish Sauce, and toss again. Mound in the center of a shallow serving dish and garnish with the reserved ingredients.

To serve: Serve with shrimp paste chips or tortilla chips, Sweet and Sour Fish Sauce (p. 47), and more thinly sliced red chile pepper.

Nutrition Information per Serving (as a main dish): 211 calories, 6 g total fat (1 g saturated fat), 63 mg cholesterol, 1253 mg sodium, 26 g carbohydrates, 4 g dietary fiber, 16 g protein

Nutrition Information per Serving (as a side dish): 106 calories, 3 g total fat (.5 g saturated fat), 31 mg cholesterol, 627 mg sodium, 13 g carbohydrates, 2 g dietary fiber, 8 g protein

Vietnamese Ginger and Pineapple Salad
(2 servings)

1/2 fresh pineapple, cut up (yields about 2 cups pineapple chunks)
1-inch piece ginger, peeled and finely minced
1/2 teaspoon salt
1/2 teaspoon sugar
5 cilantro sprigs, finely minced
1/2 red chile pepper, finely minced

1. In a large bowl, mix pineapple chunks, ginger, salt, sugar, cilantro, and chile pepper. Toss ingredients together thoroughly.

2. Refrigerate until serving time.

To serve: This refreshing salad can be served alone or to accompany any entrée.

Nutrition Information per Serving: 87 calories, 1 g total fat (0 g saturated fat), 0 mg cholesterol, 588 mg sodium, 22 g carbohydrates, 2 g dietary fiber, 1 g protein

Korean/Japanese Ginger Pickles
(30 servings)

1/4 pound fresh young ginger, peeled
1/3 cup rice vinegar
3 tablespoons sugar
1/4 teaspoon salt

1. Shave the ginger into paper-thin slices, using a sharp knife. Blanch the ginger in boiling water about 30 seconds. Drain ginger, cool, and set aside.

2. Combine vinegar, sugar and salt.

3. Add the cooled ginger to the vinegar mixture and toss well. Transfer ginger to an airtight container and refrigerate about 24 hours. Pickled ginger will keep several weeks.

To serve: Koreans and Japanese serve pickled ginger with sushi or noodles. Vietnamese add soy sauce to ginger pickles.

Nutrition Information per Serving: 7 calories, 0 g total fat (0 g saturated fat), 0 mg cholesterol, 20 mg sodium, 2 g carbohydrates, 0 g dietary fiber, 0 g protein

Vietnamese Chicken Salad

(2 main dish servings; 4 side dish servings)

1/2 pound chicken breast

1/4 head small white cabbage, shredded

1 teaspoon salt (divided)

1 tablespoon roasted sesame seeds or crushed peanuts

3 mint sprigs or 3 cilantro springs, minced

1 carrot, shredded

1 fresh red chile pepper, thinly sliced

1/2 cup Vinegar Salad Dressing (p. 57)

1-1/2 tablespoons Sweet and Sour Fish Sauce (p. 47)

1. Put chicken breasts in a medium saucepan with water to barely cover, bring to a boil, turn heat to simmer, and cook for 15 minutes, or until chicken is cooked through. Cool and shred chicken into strips.

2. In a large bowl, toss together the shredded cabbage and 1/2 teaspoon of salt. Set aside for 10 minutes. Rinse cabbage with cold water, drain, and dry.

3. Reserve some of the chicken, mint or cilantro, chile pepper, and sesame or peanuts to decorate serving dish. In a large bowl, toss together the remaining chicken, shredded cabbage, remaining salt, carrot, the remaining mint or cilantro and sesame or peanuts. Refrigerate until serving time.

4. Toss mixture with 1/2 cup Vinegar Salad Dressing (p. 57) and 1-1/2 tablespoons Sweet and Sour Fish Sauce (p. 47).

To serve: Garnish with reserved chicken, mint or cilantro, chile pepper, sesame, or peanuts. Pass the remaining Sweet and Sour Fish Sauce (p. 47) Serve with shrimp paste chips or tortilla chips. Traditionally paired with Vietnamese Chicken Rice Soup (p. 71).

Nutrition Information per Serving (as a main dish): 337 calories, 12 g total fat (3 g saturated fat), 95 mg cholesterol, 882 mg sodium, 20 g carbohydrates, 5 g dietary fiber, 37 g protein

Nutrition Information per Serving (as a side dish): 169 calories, 6 g total fat (1 g saturated fat), 48 mg cholesterol, 441 mg sodium, 10 g carbohydrates, 2 g dietary fiber, 19 g protein

Korean Sesame Cucumber Salad
(4 servings)

3 cucumbers, sliced 1/8-inch thick

1 small onion, thinly sliced

1 teaspoon salt

2 garlic cloves, finely minced

3 teaspoons sugar

3 tablespoons lemon juice

1 cayenne pepper, thinly sliced

1 tablespoon crushed, roasted sesame seeds

1/2 tablespoon sesame oil or olive oil

1. Use a food processor or a sharp knife to slice cucumbers and onion. Put cucumber in a large bowl, sprinkle with salt. Toss well, and set aside for 15 minutes.

2. Drain cucumber thoroughly and discard all liquid. Add the onion, garlic, sugar, lemon juice, cayenne pepper, sesame seeds, and sesame or olive oil. Toss well, cover, and refrigerate for 1 hour before serving.

To serve: Serve cold or at room temperature. Koreans like this salad very spicy.

Nutrition Information per Serving: 87 calories, 3 g total fat (0.4 g saturated fat), 0 mg cholesterol, 584 mg sodium, 14 g carbohydrates, 3 g dietary fiber, 3 g protein

Thai Spicy Cucumber Salad
(6 servings)

3 cucumbers, sliced 1/8-inch thick and chopped into 4 pieces
1 small onion, thinly sliced
1/4 cup rice vinegar or white vinegar
1/2 teaspoon salt
2-1/2 tablespoons sugar
1/4 cup water

Garnish:
cilantro leaves
1 cayenne pepper, thinly sliced

1. In a medium bowl, beat together the rice vinegar, salt, sugar, and water. When sugar is completely dissolved, add cucumbers, onion, and cayenne pepper. Toss well and set aside for 30 minutes.

To serve: Serve cold or at room temperature with Thai Beef Satay (p. 100) or Thai Chicken Satay (p. 84). Garnish with cilantro leaves and add cayenne pepper to taste.

Nutrition Information per Serving: 37 calories, 0 g total fat (0 g saturated fat), 0 mg cholesterol, 197 mg sodium, 9 g carbohydrates, 1 g dietary fiber, 1 g protein

Garden Salad
(2 servings)

10 sprigs cilantro
10 sprigs mint
10 sprigs basil
1/2 head lettuce, shredded
1 cup of bean sprouts
1 small cucumber, thinly sliced

To serve: Arrange all vegetables on a platter. This is a table salad and can be served with most entrées, particularly paired with Sweet and Sour Fish Sauce (p. 47).

Nutrition Information per Serving: 57 calories, 0 g total fat (0 g saturated fat), 0 mg cholesterol, 28 mg sodium, 11 g carbohydrates, 4 g dietary fiber, 4 g protein

Carrot Pickles

(10 servings)

3 carrots, shredded

1 tablespoon sugar

1/4 cup water

2 tablespoons vinegar

1/4 teaspoon salt

1. Mix carrots, sugar, water, vinegar, and salt in a medium bowl. Toss well and set aside until serving time.

To serve: These pickles go with any recipes that call for Sweet and Sour Fish Sauce (p. 47) or soy sauce.

Nutrition Information per Serving: 15 calories, 0 g total fat (0 g saturated fat), 0 mg cholesterol, 66 mg sodium, 4 g carbohydrates, 1 g dietary fiber, 0 g protein

Soups

Vietnamese Chicken Noodle Soup
(4 servings)

Broth:
1/2 small onion
1-inch piece ginger
1 pound chicken bones
8 cups water
4 pieces star anise
1/2 teaspoon salt
1/2 teaspoon sugar
1 pound chicken breasts

Noodles:
1/2 16-ounce package dry, flat rice
  noodles (pho)

Garnish:
2 scallions, thinly sliced
1 small onion, thinly sliced
5 cilantro sprigs, finely chopped
1/2 cup bean sprouts
5 sprigs basil
6 sprigs fresh culantro (ngo gai)
fresh red or green chile pepper,
  thinly sliced

Accompaniments:
lime or lemon quarters
fish sauce
hoisin sauce
hot chile sauce

1. Broil onion and ginger until charred. Using back of cleaver, smash
    the ginger and set aside.

2. Wash chicken bones; place in a medium soup pot and add water to
    cover. Bring to a boil and immediately pour off "first boiling" water
    and discard. This extra "boil up" cleanses the bones and yields a
    clearer broth. Add 8 cups of fresh water and again bring to a boil.
    Skim off foam. Add broiled onion, ginger, star anise, salt, and sugar.
    Over medium-low heat, simmer for 20 minutes.

3. Add chicken breasts and simmer until cooked through, about 15
    minutes.

4. Remove chicken breasts from broth, skin and bone if necessary, cool, and slice into 1/4-inch strips. Strain broth; discard bones and solids.

5. Soak noodles in cold water for 10 minutes. Drain. In a soup pot, bring 2 quarts fresh water to a boil. Add drained noodles and cook at a rolling boil for 7 minutes, stirring occasionally, until noodles are tender.

6. Rinse noodles under cold running water and set aside.

To serve: Divide noodles among two to four large individual serving bowls. Arrange chicken, scallions, onion, and culantro on top. Pour hot broth to cover noodles and serve immediately with garnishes and sauces. Serve with bean sprouts, basil, and chile pepper.

Nutrition Information per Serving: 321 calories, 2 g total fat (1 g saturated fat), 47 mg cholesterol, 358 mg sodium, 52 g carbohydrates, 2 g dietary fiber, 22 g protein

Vietnamese Beef Noodle Soup
(4 servings)

Broth:
1/2 small onion
1-inch piece ginger
3 pounds beef bones
10 cups water
4 pieces star anise
1/2 teaspoon salt
1/2 teaspoon sugar
1 pound lean, tender beef

Noodles:
8 ounces dry, flat rice noodles
  (pho)

Garnish:
2 scallions, thinly sliced
1 small onion, thinly sliced
5 cilantro sprigs, finely chopped
1/2 cup bean sprouts
5 sprigs basil
6 sprigs fresh culantro (ngo gai)
fresh red or green chile pepper,
  thinly sliced

Accompaniments:
lime or lemon quarters
fish sauce
hoisin sauce
hot chile sauce

1. Broil onion and ginger until charred. Using back of cleaver, smash the ginger and set aside.

2. Wash beef bones, place in a medium soup pot, and add water to cover. Bring to a boil and immediately pour off "first boiling" water and discard. This extra "boil up" cleanses the bones and yields a clearer broth. Add 10 cups of fresh water and again bring to a boil. Skim off foam. Add broiled onion, ginger, star anise, salt, and sugar. Simmer for 45 minutes over medium-low heat.

3. Slice raw beef into thin strips and set aside.

4. Remove bones from broth and strain out vegetables and seasonings.

5. Soak noodles in cold water for 10 minutes and drain. In a soup pot, bring 2 quarts of fresh water to a boil. Add drained noodles and cook 7 minutes at a rolling boil, stirring occasionally, until noodles are tender.

6. Rinse noodles under cold running water and set aside.

7. Return the broth to a boil over high heat.

To serve: Divide noodles among two to four large individual serving bowls. Arrange thinly sliced raw beef, scallions, onion, and culantro on top. Pour boiling hot broth to cover noodles and serve immediately. The boiling broth will cook the thin slices of beef. Pho is always accompanied by bean sprouts, basil leaves, culantro, and chile pepper. Serve with lime and lemon quarters, fish sauce, hoisin sauce and hot chile sauce.

Nutrition Information per Serving: 468 calories, 11 g total fat (4 g saturated fat), 98 mg cholesterol, 394 mg sodium, 52 g carbohydrates, 2 g dietary fiber, 38 g protein

Vietnamese Chicken or Duck Rice Soup with Sweet and Sour Ginger Fish Sauce

(4 servings)

1/3 cup rice
1 tablespoon oil
1 small onion, coarsely chopped
5 cups water
1-inch piece ginger, peeled,
 smashed
1/4 chicken or 2 chicken breasts
1/4 teaspoon salt

Garnish:
2 scallions, cut in 1-inch-long
 pieces
3 sprigs cilantro, finely chopped
pinch of black pepper
Sweet and Sour Ginger Fish Sauce
 (see below)

1. Wash and drain rice thoroughly. Heat the oil in a frying pan and stir-fry rice and onion until rice turns white.

2. In a soup pot, combine 5 cups of water, ginger, chicken, and salt and bring to a boil. Skim off the foam until clear and simmer until chicken is cooked through, about 15 minutes. Remove chicken from the pot and add rice and onion mixture. Simmer for 30 minutes.

3. Skin, bone, and coarsely shred the chicken and return it to the soup. If it is paired with Vietnamese Chicken Salad, reserve the chicken to make the salad. Before serving, add scallions and cilantro and sprinkle with black pepper.

To serve: This soup is paired with Vietnamese Chicken Salad (p. 62) If you prefer duck soup, substitute duck for the chicken in this recipe.

Nutrition Information per Serving (without Sweet and Sour Ginger Fish Sauce) Using Chicken : 190 calories, 5 g total fat (1 g saturated fat), 51 mg cholesterol, 214 mg sodium, 14 g carbohydrates, 1 g dietary fiber, 22 g protein

Nutrition Information per Serving (without Sweet and Sour Ginger Fish Sauce) Using Duck: 161 calories, 5 g total fat (1 g saturated fat), 68 mg cholesterol, 207 mg sodium, 14 g carbohydrates, 1 g dietary fiber, 15 g protein

Sweet and Sour Ginger Fish Sauce

Yield: 1 cup (16 tablespoons; 2 tablespoons per serving)

2 garlic cloves, finely minced

1-inch piece ginger, peeled and minced

3 tablespoons sugar

2 tablespoons lime or lemon juice

1/2 cup warm water

6 tablespoons fish sauce

1/2 teaspoon ground red chile pepper, or to taste

1. In a small bowl mix the minced garlic, ginger, sugar, lime or lemon juice, water, and fish sauce until the sugar has completely dissolved. Add ground red chile pepper to taste.

Nutrition Information per Serving: 26 calories, 0 g total fat (0 g saturated fat), 0 mg cholesterol, 1043 mg sodium, 6 g carbohydrates, 0 g dietary fiber, 1 g protein

Thai Coconut Chicken Soup
(4 servings)

1-1/2 cups water

1 cup coconut milk (divided)

1/2 pound chicken breast, diced

5 slices galanga (available in Asian grocery stores, particularly Thai, Vietnamese, or Korean) or ginger

2 tablespoons fish sauce or 3/4 teaspoon salt

1 3-inch stalk lemongrass, smashed

1 fresh red chile pepper

2 bergamot leaves or 1 teaspoon lime zest, finely shredded

lemon juice

fish sauce

Garnish:

1 scallion, thinly sliced

1 fresh red chile pepper, thinly sliced

1. Smash the lemongrass and cut it into 1-inch pieces.

2. In a medium saucepan, bring water to a boil. Add 1/2 cup of the coconut milk, chicken, galanga, fish sauce, and lemongrass. Simmer until chicken is cooked through, about 15 minutes.

3. Add the remaining 1/2 cup of coconut milk, the whole red chile pepper, and the bergamot leaves or lime zest. Stir and immediately remove from the heat.

To serve: Serve with lemon juice and fish sauce to taste. Garnish with scallions and additional red chile pepper.

Nutrition Information per Serving: 108 calories, 2 g total fat (1 g saturated fat), 44 mg cholesterol, 764 mg sodium, 4 g carbohydrates, 1 g dietary fiber, 18 g protein

Thai Hot and Sour Shrimp Soup
(4 servings)

1 3-inch stalk fresh lemongrass

3 slices galanga, (available in Asian grocery stores, particularly Thai, Vietnamese, or Korean)

2 Kaffir lime leaves (Thai lime leaves) or 1 teaspoon grated lemon zest

1 teaspoon oil

1 garlic clove, finely minced

1/2 teaspoon dry red pepper or 1 fresh cayenne pepper, finely minced

3 cups chicken stock or 3 cups water and 1/2 teaspoon salt

2 tablespoons fish sauce or 1/2 teaspoon salt

3 tablespoons fresh lime juice or to taste

1/2 teaspoon sugar

8 fresh mushrooms, thinly sliced

10 medium shrimp, shelled and deveined

Garnish:

1 fresh red chile pepper, thinly sliced

4 sprigs cilantro

1. Smash lemongrass and cut into 1-inch pieces.

2. In a medium saucepan, heat oil and sauté garlic until fragrant. Quickly stir in red pepper. Add lemongrass, lime leaves and chicken stock. Bring to a boil, skim off foam. Lower heat and simmer about 10 minutes. Add fish sauce or salt, lime juice, sugar, and fresh mushrooms. Remove from heat until serving time.

To serve: Before serving, return the broth to a boil and drop in shrimp; cook for 3 minutes, until pink and curled. Garnish with sliced red chile pepper and cilantro leaves.

Nutrition Information per Serving: 61 calories, 2 g total fat (0.4 g saturated fat), 23 mg cholesterol, 1,198 mg sodium, 7 g carbohydrates, 1 g dietary fiber, 5 g protein. If using Chicken Broth recipes (p. 80), sodium is 811 mg per serving.

Vietnamese Chicken or Shrimp Pineapple Soup

(4 servings)

1/4 cup warm water
1 tablespoon tamarind pulp
1 teaspoon oil
2 garlic cloves, minced
1/2 fresh pineapple, cored and
    thinly sliced or 1 can sugar-free
    pineapple chunks
1 teaspoon sugar
4 cups water
10 medium shrimp, shelled and
    deveined or 1/2 pound chicken
    breast

1 tomato, cut into 8 pieces
2 tablespoons fish sauce or 1/2
    teaspoon salt

Garnish:
1 scallion, sliced
5 sprigs rau om (Vietnamese herb)
    or culantro or cilantro
1 red chile pepper, thinly sliced

1. In a small bowl, mix warm water and tamarind pulp. Mash tamarind with a small spoon to extract as much tamarind juice as possible. Set aside.

2. In a small soup pot, heat oil and sauté minced garlic until brown. Stir in pineapple and sugar. Add 4 cups water and bring to a boil.

3. Add tamarind mixture, shrimp, tomato, and fish sauce or salt. Skim off foam and simmer for 5 minutes.

To serve: Garnish with scallions; rau om, culantro, or cilantro; and sliced red chile pepper.

Nutrition Information per Serving Using Chicken: 131 calories, 2 g total fat (0.4 g saturated fat), 33 mg cholesterol, 311 mg sodium, 14 g carbohydrates, 2 g dietary fiber, 14 g protein

Nutrition Information per Serving Using Shrimp: 85 calories, 2 g total fat (0.3 g saturated fat), 23 mg cholesterol, 296 mg sodium, 14 g carbohydrates, 2 g dietary fiber, 4 g protein

Japanese Miso Soup

(4 servings)

1 4-inch x 6-inch block soft tofu

4 cups water

2 teaspoons dashi (nomoto), a powdered soup stock available at Korean
  grocery stores

6 fresh mushrooms, sliced

3 tablespoons miso paste (adjust to taste)

2 scallions, finely chopped

ground black pepper, to taste

1. Divide tofu into 8 pieces. In a medium soup pot, mix 4 cups water
    and dashi. Bring to a boil.

2. Add tofu and mushrooms and simmer about 3 minutes. Add miso
    paste and gently dissolve completely. Immediately turn off the heat.

To serve: Reheat soup and add scallions. Pour into small bowls and sprinkle with ground
black pepper.

Nutrition Information per Serving: 150 calories, 8 g total fat (1 g saturated fat), 0 mg cholesterol, 491 mg sodium, 8 g carbohydrates, 3 g dietary fiber, 15 g protein

Vietnamese Clear Vegetable Soup
(4 servings)

8 medium shrimp or 1/2 cup of lean ground meat (pork, beef, or turkey)
1/4 teaspoon sugar
1/4 teaspoon salt
1/4 teaspoon black pepper
3 cups vegetables (broccoli, watercress, cabbage, spinach—choose your
   favorites)
3 cups water
1-1/2 tablespoons fish sauce or 1/4 teaspoon salt

Garnish:
5 cilantro sprigs, finely chopped
2 scallions, thinly sliced
pinch of black pepper

1. If using shrimp, shell and devein. Use back of cleaver to smash
    shrimp, then finely mince to a paste. Mix in sugar, salt, and pepper.

2. If using ground meat, just mix in sugar, salt and pepper.

3. Wash and coarsely chop the vegetables. Set aside.

4. In a medium soup pot, bring water to a boil, add shrimp (or pork, beef,
    or turkey) paste a teaspoon at a time. Skim foam until broth is clear.
    Add vegetables and cook 2 minutes, then add fish sauce or salt.

To serve: Transfer soup to a large bowl. Garnish soup with cilantro, sliced scallions, and an additional pinch of pepper.

Nutrition Information per Serving Using Shrimp: 29 calories, 0 g total fat (0 g saturated fat), 18 mg cholesterol, 707 mg sodium, 3 g carbohydrates, 1 g dietary fiber, 4 g protein

Nutrition Information per Serving Using Pork: 91 calories, 6 g total fat (2 g saturated fat), 20 mg cholesterol, 705 mg sodium, 3 g carbohydrates, 1 g dietary fiber, 6 g protein

Nutrition Information per Serving Using Beef: 82 calories, 5 g total fat (2 g saturated fat), 20 mg cholesterol, 708 mg sodium, 3 g carbohydrates, 1 g dietary fiber, 7 g protein

Nutrition Information per Serving Using Turkey: 58 calories, 3 g total fat (1 g saturated fat), 22 mg cholesterol, 716 mg sodium, 3 g carbohydrates, 1 g dietary fiber, 6 g protein

Beef Broth

(10 servings; 1 cup per serving)

4 pounds beef bones

18 cups water

1 1-inch piece ginger, peeled and smashed

1 large onion, quartered

1 teaspoon salt

1 teaspoon sugar

1. Wash beef bones, place in a medium soup pot, and add water to cover. Bring to a boil and immediately pour off "first boiling" water and discard. This extra "boil up" cleanses the bones and yields a clearer broth. Add 18 cups of fresh water and again bring to a boil. Skim off foam. Add onion, ginger, salt, and sugar. Over medium-low heat, simmer for 2 hours.

2. Remove bones from broth and strain out vegetables and seasonings. Set aside until cool.

3. Transfer to small containers and freeze for later use. Before using, defrost broth completely at room temperature.

To serve: Serve as a side dish with any entrée.

Nutrition Information per Cup: 14 calories, 0 g total fat (0 g saturated fat), 0 mg cholesterol, 251 mg sodium, 3 g carbohydrates, 1 g dietary fiber, 0 g protein

Chicken Broth

(10 serving; 1 cup per serving)

4 pounds chicken bones
15 cups water
1 large onion, quartered
1 teaspoon salt
1 teaspoon sugar

1. Wash chicken bones, place in a medium soup pot, and add water to cover. Bring to a boil and immediately pour off "first boiling" water and discard. This extra "boil up" cleanses the bones and yields a clearer broth. Add 15 cups of fresh water and again bring to a boil. Skim off foam. Add onion, salt, and sugar. Over medium-low heat, simmer for 1 hour.

2. Proceed as for Beef Broth.

To serve: Serve as a side dish with any entrée.

Nutrition Information per Cup: 14 calories, 0 g total fat (0 g saturated fat), 0 mg cholesterol, 249 mg sodium, 3 g carbohydrates, 1 g dietary fiber, 0 g protein

Vegetable Broth
(12 servings; 1 cup per serving)

5 carrots, cut into 3-inch lengths

1/2 head cabbage, coarsely chopped

5 celery stalks, cut into 3-inch lengths

15 cups water

1 large onion, quartered

1 teaspoon salt

1 teaspoon sugar

1. Wash carrots, cabbage, and celery stalks. In a medium soup pot, add 15 cups of fresh water and bring all the ingredients to a boil. Skim off foam. Add onion, salt, and sugar. Over medium-low heat, simmer for 1 hour.

2. Remove vegetables from broth and proceed as for Beef Broth.

To serve: Serve as a side dish with any entrée.

Nutrition Information per Cup: 36 calories, 0 g total fat (0 g saturated fat), 0 mg cholesterol, 234 mg sodium, 8 g carbohydrates, 3 g dietary fiber, 1 g protein

Main Dishes

Poultry

Chinese Chicken on Chicken-Flavored Rice with Sweet Ginger Soy Sauce
(4 servings)

6 cups water
1-inch piece ginger, peeled and smashed
1/2 teaspoon salt
1/4 teaspoon sugar
1 pound chicken breasts
4 servings Chicken-Flavored Rice (p. 42)
Sweet Ginger Soy Sauce (see below)

Garnish:
5 cilantro sprigs, finely chopped
2 scallions, thinly sliced
pinch of black pepper

1. In a large saucepan, bring 6 cups of water to a boil. Add chicken breasts, ginger, salt, and sugar and simmer until cooked through, about 15 minutes.

2. Remove chicken breasts from broth. When cooled, bone and cut chicken into small pieces. Reserve the broth to cook rice and the remaining broth for soup.

3. Prepare Sweet Ginger Soy Sauce (facing page).

To serve: Arrange chicken on a serving plate. Serve chicken with Chinese Chicken-Flavored Rice (p. 42) accompanied with Sweet Ginger Soy Sauce (below). It can be paired with Chinese Cabbage Pickles (p. 53), Korean Kimchee (p. 54), Korean/Japanese Ginger Pickles (p. 61), and/or Korean Sesame (p. 63) or Thai Spicy (p. 64) cucumber salad. Vietnamese serve this dish with a large bowl of Chicken Broth. Transfer hot chicken broth to a large bowl and add cilantro and sliced scallions. Sprinkle with a pinch of black pepper.

Nutrition Information per Serving (for chicken only): 140 calories, 5 g total fat (2 g saturated fat), 54 mg cholesterol, 349 mg sodium, 2 g carbohydrates, 0 g dietary fiber, 20 g protein

Sweet Ginger Soy Sauce
Yield: 3/4 cup (1 tablespoon per serving)

2 garlic cloves, finely minced

2 tablespoons honey

8 tablespoons soy sauce

2 tablespoons warm water

1/2 teaspoon oil (optional)

1 tablespoon fresh ginger, peeled and finely minced

1 teaspoon ground red pepper or red chile paste (optional)

1. In a small bowl, beat together garlic, honey, soy sauce, warm water, oil, and ginger. Stir in ground red pepper or red chile paste to taste.

To serve: Serve with any meat entrée.

Nutrition Information per Serving with Oil: 21 calories, 0 g total fat (0 g saturated fat), 0 mg cholesterol, 614 mg sodium, 3 g carbohydrates, 0 g dietary fiber, 1 g protein

Nutrition Information per Serving without Oil: 19 calories, 0 g total fat (0 g saturated fat), 0 mg cholesterol, 614 mg sodium, 3 g carbohydrates, 0 g dietary fiber, 1 g protein

Thai Chicken Satay
(2 main dish servings; 4 side dish servings)

2 tablespoons unsweetened coconut milk

1/2 teaspoon sugar

2 garlic cloves, finely minced

1/2 teaspoon curry powder

1/2 teaspoon cornstarch

1 tablespoon fish sauce or 1/2 teaspoon salt

1 tablespoon lime or lemon juice

1 teaspoon oil

8 ounces boneless chicken breast, cut into 1-inch x 2-inch strips

8 bamboo skewers, soaked in water for at least 10 minutes

1. In a large bowl, mix together coconut milk, sugar, garlic, curry powder, cornstarch, fish sauce or salt, lime or lemon juice, and oil. Marinate chicken in this mixture for 20 minutes.

2. Thread marinated chicken onto skewers. Place chicken skewers on the grill, turning and brushing occasionally with the marinade, until they turn golden. If cooking indoors, broil chicken skewers for 3 minutes, turning them frequently and brushing meat with the remaining marinade.

To serve: Serve with Thai Spicy Cucumber Salad (p. 64) and Thai Peanut Sauce (p. 101). This can be an appetizer or a main dish.

Nutrition Information per Serving (as a main dish): 164 calories, 4 g total fat (1 g saturated fat), 66 mg cholesterol, 776 mg sodium, 4 g carbohydrates, 0 g dietary fiber, 27 g protein

Nutrition Information per Serving (as an appetizer): 82 calories, 2 g total fat (0.4 g saturated fat), 33 mg cholesterol, 388 mg sodium, 2 g carbohydrates, 0 g dietary fiber, 13 g protein

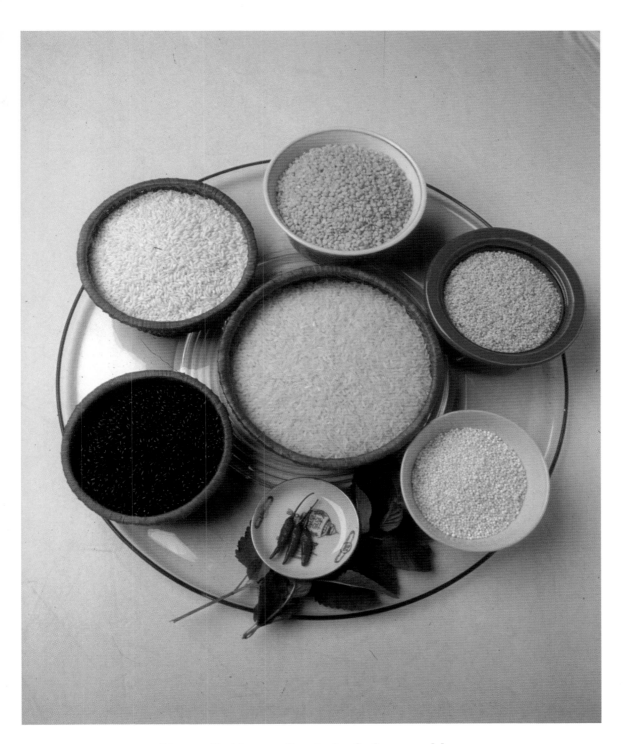

Essential ingredients in Asian cooking

These can easily be found in supermarkets or in Asian grocery stores. Clockwise from top: dried yellow mung beans, roasted white sesame (in red bowl), tapioca pearls, fresh red Thai chile peppers (in small dish), mint sprigs (tucked under dish), black rice, sweet rice (also called sticky or glutinous rice). Center: long-grain white rice.

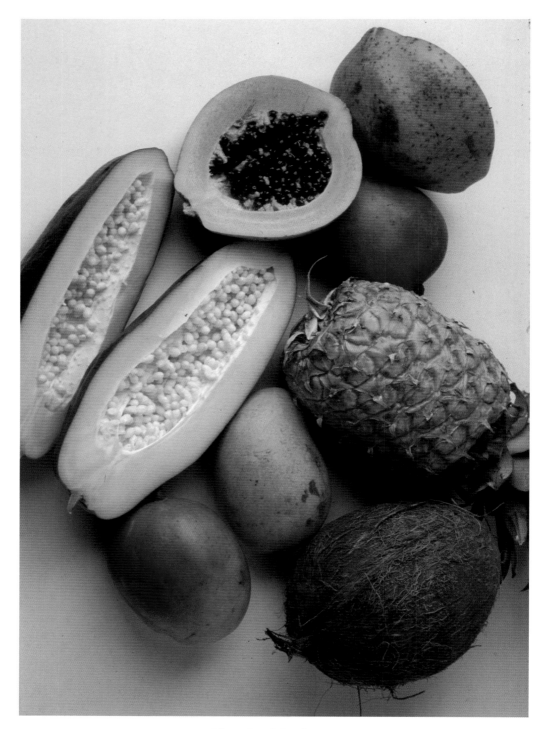

Tropical fruits

Tropical fruits are available in most local supermarkets. Green papaya and green mango make delightful salads. Ripe papaya and ripe mangos are delicious for desserts and fruit shakes. Clockwise from top: Ripe papaya (cut in halves), mango, pineapple, whole dry coconut, two kinds of mangos, green papaya (cut in halves).

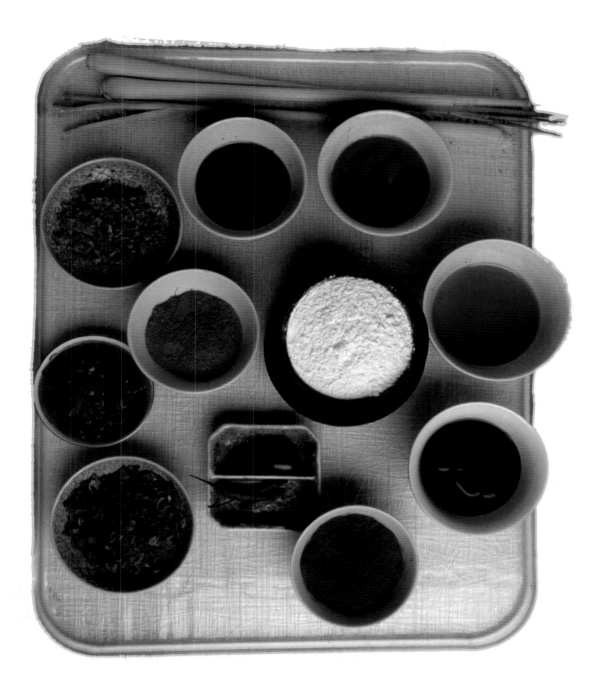

Characteristic components in Asian cuisine

Top: fresh lemongrass. Outer circle of ingredients, clockwise from upper right: red chile sauce, fish sauce, hoisin sauce, five-spice powder, dried fried shallots, red chile pepper paste, dried minced cabbage, soy sauce. Inner circle of ingredients, clockwise: red and green Thai chile peppers (in the square dish), curry powder, tapioca starch.

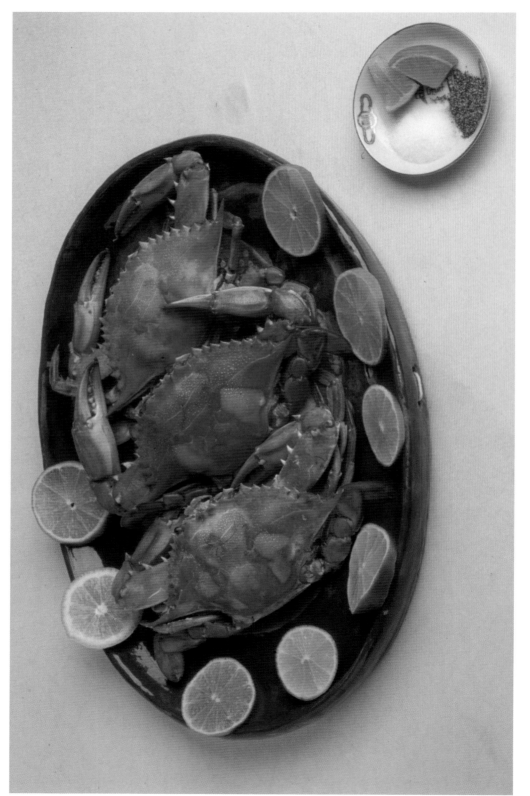

Crabs in beer

Fish and seafood play an important role in the Asian diet. Most Asians love steamed crabs. Seafood is easy and fast to cook, and it is healthier than meat. Fresh seafood is readily available at local markets.

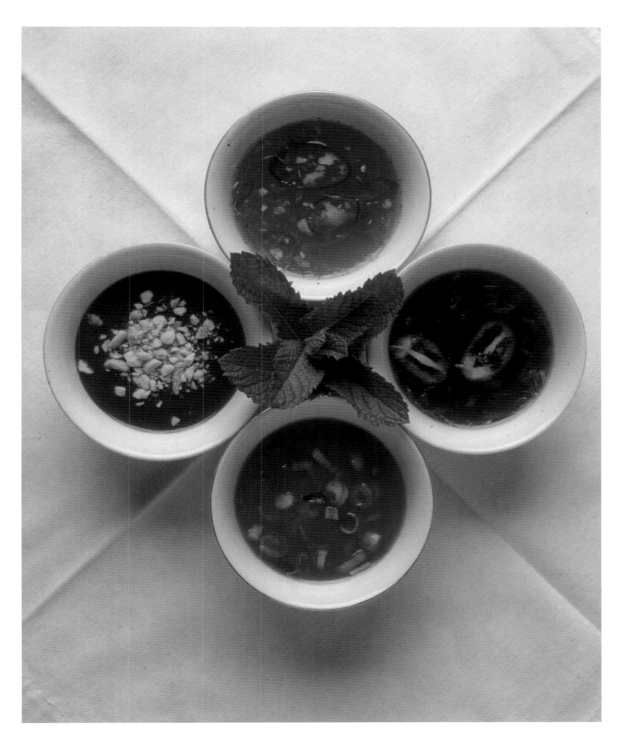

Sauces

A variety of sauces accompany every Asian meal. Sweet and Sour Fish Sauce or Sweet and Sour Soy Sauce can be served with any entrée. Raw Fish Sauce and Soy Sauce from the bottle can be served plain or cooked. Clockwise from top: Sweet and Sour Fish Sauce, Sweet and Sour Soy Sauce, Sweet and Sour Tomato Sauce, Peanut Hoisin Sauce.

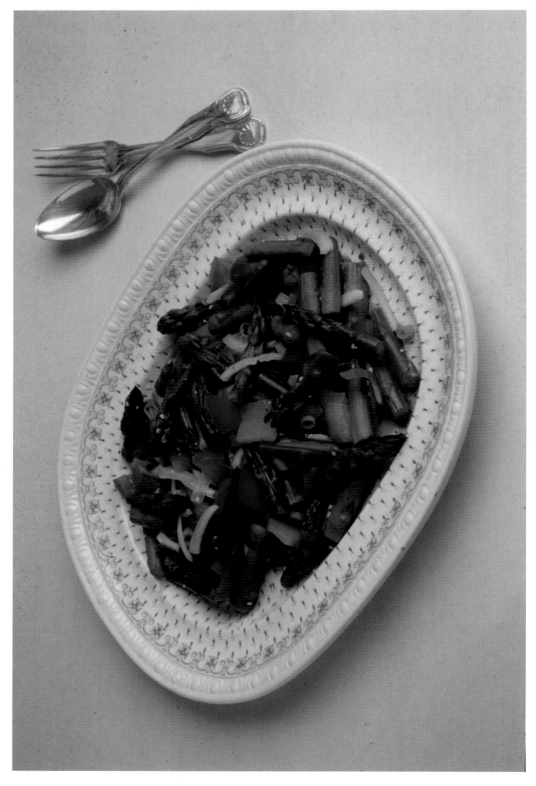

Asparagus Salad

Vegetables are a major part of an Asian meal. A combination of abundant herbs and vegetables makes an appealing meal. Asparagus salad, in particular, is one of my favorites. It is a delicious dish, fast and easy to prepare.

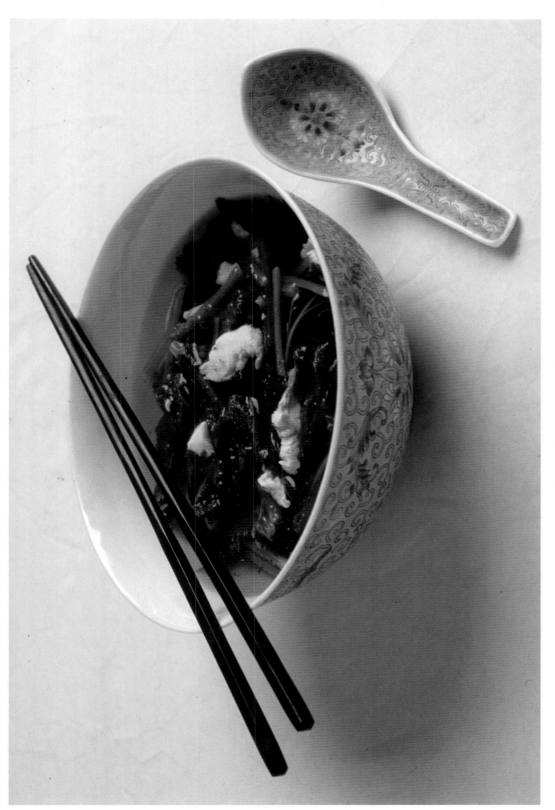

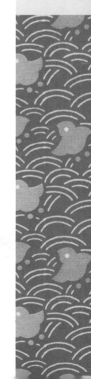

Clear Vegetable Soup

Soup is one of the three courses in the daily dinner of Asian families, especially the Vietnamese and Chinese. Clear Vegetable Soup is light and low fat and makes a delicious diet dish.

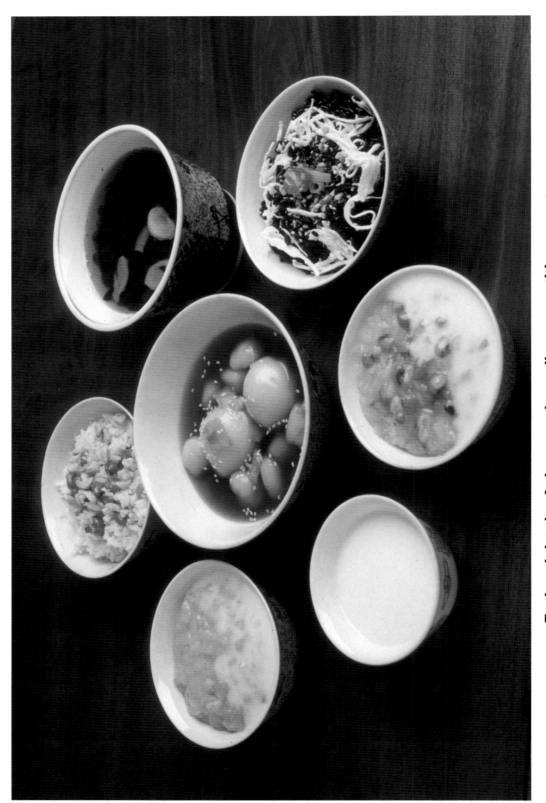

Eating right the Asian way does allow something sweet.

In Saigon vendors would walk along the streets calling out these delicious desserts for sale in the baskets they carry on a pole across their shoulders. Clockwise from upper left: Peanut Sticky Rice, Chinese Black-Eyed Peas in Ginger and Orange-Flavored Sauce, Black Rice with Shredded Coconut, Black-Eyed Peas Pudding in Coconut Milk, Coconut Sauce, Corn Pudding with Coconut Milk. Center: Mung Bean Rice Balls in Brown Sugar Syrup.

Japanese Chicken Teriyaki
(4 servings)

5 tablespoons teriyaki sauce or soy sauce

2 tablespoons red wine

2 tablespoons honey or brown sugar

1/2 teaspoon ground ginger or 1 tablespoon fresh ginger,
   peeled and finely minced

1 pound chicken breast

1 tablespoon roasted, unsalted sesame seeds

2 garlic cloves, finely minced

1 small onion, thinly sliced

1 teaspoon oil

pinch black pepper

1. In medium bowl, beat together teriyaki or soy sauce, wine, honey or brown sugar, and ginger. Marinate chicken in the mixture for 15 minutes.

2. Heat the oil in a frying pan until hot. Sauté garlic and onion until soft, about 5 minutes. Add marinated chicken and teriyaki or soy sauce mixture. Simmer about 10 minutes or until chicken is cooked through.

To serve: Transfer chicken onto a serving plate. Sprinkle sesame seeds and a pinch of black pepper.

Nutrition Information per Serving: 213 calories, 4 g total fat (1 g saturated fat), 66 mg cholesterol, 939 mg sodium, 15 g carbohydrates, 1 g dietary fiber, 28 g protein

Vietnamese Ginger Chicken

(4 servings)

1 pound boneless chicken breasts, cut into small cubes

2 teaspoons honey

1/2 teaspoon salt

1/2 teaspoon black pepper

1 teaspoon cornstarch

1 tablespoon oil

2 cloves garlic, finely minced

1 1/2-inch piece ginger, peeled and finely chopped

1/3 cup water

2 tablespoons fish sauce or soy sauce

1/2 small onion, chopped

3 scallions, chopped

freshly ground black pepper

1. Marinate chicken in a mixture of honey, salt, pepper, and cornstarch for 15 minutes.

2. Heat the oil in the fry pan until hot. Sauté garlic until golden. Add marinated chicken and ginger and stir until the mixture browns. Add water and fish or soy sauce and simmer 10 minutes. Add chopped onions and scallions. Simmer about 5 minutes, stirring occasionally, until caramel brown.

To serve: Sprinkle with black pepper to taste and serve hot with rice.

Nutrition Information per Serving: 180 calories, 5 g total fat (1 g saturated fat), 66 mg cholesterol, 1062 mg sodium, 6 g carbohydrates, 0 g dietary fiber, 27 g protein

Chinese Chicken with Mustard Greens
(*4 servings*)

1 pound boneless chicken breasts

8 black Chinese mushrooms, soaked

2 pounds mustard greens

1/2 teaspoon salt

1/2 teaspoon black pepper

1/4 teaspoon sugar

1 teaspoon oil

1 cup chicken broth

1 teaspoon cornstarch

1/2-inch piece ginger, peeled and finely chopped

3 tablespoons oyster sauce

2 tablespoons soy sauce

freshly ground black pepper

1. Put chicken breasts in a medium saucepan, barely cover with water, bring to a boil, turn heat down to simmer, and cook uncovered for 15 minutes, or until chicken is cooked through. Cool and shred chicken into coarse strips. Reserve broth for sauce.

2. Soak Chinese black mushrooms overnight. Discard hard stems and set aside.

3. Wash mustard greens thoroughly. Discard the tough stems and cut the greens into 2-inch pieces. In a medium saucepan, bring water to cover to a boil and add salt. Blanch mustard greens about 1 minute. Rinse in cold water and drain thoroughly.

4. In a large bowl, toss the chicken, mustard greens, mushrooms, salt, pepper, sugar, and oil thoroughly. Arrange shredded chicken, mustard greens, and mushrooms in a deep baking dish.

5. Combine 1 cup of chicken broth, cornstarch, ginger, oyster sauce, and soy sauce in a small saucepan. Cook over low heat. Stir constantly until the mixture is thick and clear.

6. Pour sauce over chicken and greens. Put the baking dish in a steamer and steam for 15 minutes. If you're using a microwave, cover the dish and steam for 3 minutes.

To serve: Transfer to a deep serving plate. Arrange black mushrooms around plate. Pour sauce over chicken and greens. Sprinkle with black pepper and serve hot.

Nutrition Information per Serving: 228 calories, 3 g total fat (1 g saturated fat), 66 mg cholesterol, 994 mg sodium, 19 g carbohydrates, 9 g dietary fiber, 34 g protein

Indian Chicken Curry
(6 servings)

2 teaspoons salt

1/2 teaspoon crushed red pepper

1 tablespoon sugar

3 tablespoons curry powder

3 tablespoons tomato paste

1 pound boneless chicken breasts, cut into bite-size pieces

2 tablespoons oil

3 garlic cloves, finely minced

1 small onion, coarsely chopped

1 stalk lemongrass, finely chopped

1 cup water

1 cup 2% milk

1 cup coconut milk

1 medium sweet potato, peeled and cut into large dice

1 white potato, peeled and cut into large dice

1. In a large bowl, thoroughly mix salt, crushed red pepper, sugar, curry powder, and tomato paste. Coat chicken with this mixture and marinate for 10 minutes.

2. Heat oil in a deep pot and stir-fry the garlic, onion, and lemongrass until fragrant. Add chicken and stir-fry about 5 minutes more. Pour water, milk, and coconut milk into the pan, stir in sweet potato, white potato, and simmer for 20 minutes.

To serve: Indian curry is more often hot than not. Serve this dish with French bread, as we do in Vietnam or, if you prefer, with rice.

Nutrition Information per Serving: 227 calories, 7 g total fat (1 g saturated fat), 47 mg cholesterol, 876 mg sodium, 20 g carbohydrates, 2 g dietary fiber, 21 g protein

Vietnamese Chicken Ragout
(6 servings)

1 teaspoon salt

1 teaspoon sugar

3 tablespoons tomato paste

1 pound boneless chicken breasts, cut into bite-size pieces

1 tablespoon oil

2 garlic cloves, finely minced

1 medium onion, coarsely chopped

4 cups water

1/2 cup red wine

1 medium potato, peeled and cut into large dice

1/2 cup green peas

1 cup white mushrooms, cut in half

1. In a large bowl, thoroughly mix salt, sugar, and tomato paste. Coat chicken with this mixture and marinate for 15 minutes.

2. Heat oil in a deep pot and stir-fry the garlic and onion until fragrant. Add chicken and sauté about 5 more minutes. Pour water and red wine into the pan, stir in potatoes, green peas, and mushrooms, and simmer for 20 minutes.

To serve: Serve with French bread or rice.

Nutrition Information per Serving: 158 calories, 3 g total fat (1 g saturated fat), 44 mg cholesterol, 449 mg sodium, 9 g carbohydrates, 1 g dietary fiber, 19 g protein

Pork/Beef

Vietnamese Pineapple Caramel Pork
(6 servings)

1 pound boneless pork, cut into small cubes
3 tablespoons caramel sauce (see below)
1/2 teaspoon salt
1/2 teaspoon black pepper
1 tablespoon oil
2 garlic cloves, finely minced
1/4 pineapple, cored and cut into chunks or 1 cup sugar-free
   chunk pineapple
4 cups water
5 tablespoons fish sauce or soy sauce
1/2 small onion, chopped
3 scallions, chopped
freshly ground black pepper

Caramel Sauce:
3 tablespoons sugar
3 tablespoons water
1/4 cup warm water

1. For the caramel sauce, combine 3 tablespoons sugar and 3 table-
    spoons water in a medium-small nonstick saucepan, and bring it to a
    boil. Turn the heat down to medium low and stir continuously until
    the mixture turns caramel brown. Add 1/4 cup warm water and con-
    tinue to stir until it becomes a brown syrup.

2. Marinate pork in a mixture of the caramel, salt, and pepper for 15
    minutes.

3. Heat the oil in a medium saucepan and sauté the garlic until fra-
    grant. Stir-fry the marinated pork about 10 minutes. Add pineapple

chunks, water, and fish or soy sauce. Bring the mixture to a boil and skim off foam. Reduce heat to medium low and simmer 30 minutes more. Add onions and scallions. Simmer about another 10 minutes over medium-low heat, stirring occasionally, until caramel brown.

To serve: Sprinkle with black pepper to taste and serve hot with Asian Plain Rice (p. 36).

Nutrition Information per Serving: 167 calories, 7 g total fat (2 g saturated fat), 46 mg cholesterol, 1401 mg sodium, 9 g carbohydrates, 1 g dietary fiber, 17 g protein

Thai Pork in Spicy Basil Sauce
(6 servings)

1 pound boneless pork, cut into thin bite-size slices
1 tablespoon oyster sauce
1/2 teaspoon cornstarch
1 teaspoon honey
1/2 teaspoon salt
1/2 teaspoon black pepper
1 tablespoon oil
2 cloves garlic, finely minced
1/3 cup water
2 tablespoons fish sauce
1/2 small onion, chopped
3 scallions, chopped
5 sprigs basil
1 red chile pepper, finely chopped
freshly ground black pepper

1. Marinate pork in a mixture of oyster sauce, cornstarch, honey, salt, and pepper for 15 minutes.

2. Heat the oil in the fry pan until hot. Sauté the garlic until golden. Stir-fry marinated pork until it has browned. Add water and fish sauce and simmer 8 minutes. Add onions, chopped scallions, fresh basil leaves, and red chile pepper and simmer about another 5 minutes, stirring occasionally, until caramel brown.

To serve: Sprinkle with black pepper to taste and serve hot with Asian Plain Rice (p. 36).

Nutrition Information per Serving: 146 calories, 7 g total fat (2 g saturated fat), 46 mg cholesterol, 564 mg sodium, 3 g carbohydrates, 1 g dietary fiber, 17 g protein

Vietnamese Five-Spice Pork Chops
(4 servings)

1 tablespoon fish sauce

1 tablespoon oyster sauce

1 tablespoon honey

1/2 teaspoon salt

1 teaspoon five-spice powder

1/2 teaspoon freshly ground black pepper

1/2 teaspoon sugar

1/2 teaspoon cornstarch

2 garlic cloves, finely minced

4 boneless, thin cut pork chops

1. Combine fish sauce, oyster sauce, honey, salt, five-spice powder, pepper, sugar, cornstarch, and garlic in a large bowl. Marinate pork chops in this mixture about 30 minutes.

2. Preheat oven to 375 degrees. Arrange pork chops on a baking sheet and bake 15 minutes, turning occasionally.

3. Turn on broiler and broil on each side for 5 minutes. Watch carefully to avoid burning.

To serve: Serve with Asian Plain Rice (p. 36), Vietnamese Tomato Rice (p. 37), or Vietnamese Lemon Rice (p. 38).

Nutrition Information per Serving: 137 calories, 4 g total fat (1 g saturated fat), 54 mg cholesterol, 492 mg sodium, 7g carbohydrates, 0 g dietary fiber, 18 g protein

Vietnamese Pan-Fried Lemongrass Pork or Beef
(6 servings)

1 pound boneless pork, thinly sliced, or 1 pound tender beef sirloin, thinly sliced

1 tablespoon oyster sauce

1/2 teaspoon cornstarch

1/2 teaspoon salt

1/2 teaspoon sugar

1/2 teaspoon black pepper

1 tablespoon oil

2 garlic cloves, finely minced

1/2 small onion, thickly sliced

1 stalk lemongrass, tender portion finely chopped

1 hot red chile pepper, minced

2 tablespoons fish sauce

freshly ground black pepper

1. Marinate pork or sirloin slices in a mixture of oyster sauce, cornstarch, salt, sugar, and pepper for 15 minutes.

2. Heat the oil in a fry pan over medium-high heat until hot. Sauté garlic and onion until fragrant. Add lemongrass and red pepper and stir for 1 minute. Add marinated meat and sauté until browned. Add fish sauce and stir another 5 minutes.

To serve: Sprinkle with black pepper to taste and serve hot with rice, a vegetable side dish, and clear soup.

Nutrition Information per Serving Using Pork: 142 calories, 7 g total fat (2 g saturated fat), 46 mg cholesterol, 430 mg sodium, 3 g carbohydrates, 0 g dietary fiber, 16 g protein

Nutrition Information per Serving Using Beef: 189 calories, 12 g total fat (4 g saturated fat), 50 mg cholesterol, 428 mg sodium, 3 g carbohydrates, 0 g dietary fiber, 15 g protein

Vietnamese Barbecued Lemongrass Pork or Beef on Rice Vermicelli

(4 servings)

1 pound boneless pork, thinly sliced, or 1 pound tender
  beef sirloin, thinly sliced
1 tablespoon oyster sauce
1/2 teaspoon cornstarch
1/2 teaspoon salt
1/2 teaspoon black pepper
1/2 teaspoon sugar
1 tablespoon oil
2 garlic cloves, finely chopped
1/2 small onion, finely chopped
1 stalk lemongrass, tender portion finely chopped
freshly ground black pepper
8 bamboo skewers, soaked in warm water for at least 10 minutes
1/2 pound rice vermicelli
Garden Salad (p. 65)
Carrot Pickles (p. 66)
1 tablespoon crushed peanuts
Sweet and Sour Fish Sauce (p. 47)
1 hot red chile pepper, minced

Garnish:
5 sprigs fresh cilantro, chopped
5 sprigs fresh basil, chopped
5 sprigs fresh mint, chopped

1. Proceed as for the Vietnamese Pan-Fried Lemongrass Pork or Beef, but omit the 2 tablespoons of fish sauce.

2. If you prefer barbecued pork or beef, thread marinated pork onto skewers, leaving 2 inches free at each end. Place pork or beef skewers on the grill, brushing them occasionally with the marinade and turning occasionally until they turn golden brown. You may also grill indoors under an oven broiler.

3. Prepare Garden Salad (p. 65).

4. Prepare Carrot Pickles (p. 66).

5. Prepare Rice Vermicelli (see below).

6. Prepare Sweet and Sour Fish Sauce (p. 47).

To serve: Prepare four large bowls lined with Garden Salad and chopped herbs. Divide Rice Vermicelli among four bowls. Strip barbecued pork or beef from skewers and place on top of Rice Vermicelli and sprinkle with crushed peanuts. Serve immediately accompanied by 3 tablespoons of Sweet and Sour Fish Sauce per bowl (p. 47), Carrot Pickles (p. 66), and hot chile pepper.

Nutrition Information per Serving Using Pork: 209 calories, 10 g total fat (3 g saturated fat), 69 mg cholesterol, 384 mg sodium, 4 g carbohydrates, 0 g dietary fiber, 24 g protein

Nutrition Information per Serving Using Beef: 278 calories, 19 g total fat (7 g saturated fat), 75 mg cholesterol, 381 mg sodium, 4 g carbohydrates, 0 g dietary fiber, 23 g protein

Rice Vermicelli

(4 servings)

1/2 pound rice vermicelli

1. In a deep pot, bring 2 quarts of water to a boil. Add rice vermicelli and stir gently until vermicelli is clear white and soft, about 5 minutes. Rinse under cold running water, drain thoroughly, and set aside.

To serve: Rice Vermicelli can be served with any entrée, accompanied by Sweet and Sour Fish Sauce (p. 47) and Garden Salad (p. 65). Can also be served with Indian Chicken Curry (p. 89), Vietnamese Chicken or Shrimp Sweet and Sour Pineapple Soup (p. 75), or Vietnamese Catfish on Dill (p. 110).

Nutrition Information per Serving: 206 calories, 0 g total fat (0 g saturated fat), 0 mg cholesterol, 103 mg sodium, 47 g carbohydrates, 1 g dietary fiber, 2 g protein

Korean Barbecued Beef
(4 servings)

1 pound tender beef sirloin, cut into 1/2-inch-thick pieces
1/2 tablespoon sugar
1/2 teaspoon black pepper
2 garlic cloves, finely minced
1/2 tablespoon honey
1 tablespoon ginger, peeled and finely minced
2 scallions, thinly sliced
1 teaspoon sesame oil
1 tablespoon unsalted sesame seeds, roasted

1. Use a sharp knife to cut a crisscross pattern in the meat.

2. In a large bowl, mix together the sugar, pepper, garlic, honey, ginger, scallions, sesame oil, and sesame seeds. Marinate the meat in this mixture for 1 hour.

3. Preheat oven to 375 degrees. Bake marinated beef for 15 minutes, turning occasionally. Turn oven to broil and broil the meat for 5 minutes, turning frequently to avoid burning.

To serve: Serve with Asian Plain Rice (p. 36), Kimchee (p. 54), Korean Cucumber Salad (p. 63), or Chinese Cabbage Pickles (p. 53).

Nutrition Information per Serving: 272 calories, 17 g total fat (6 g saturated fat), 75 mg cholesterol, 63 mg sodium, 6 g carbohydrates, 1 g dietary fiber, 23 g protein

Thai Beef Satay
(2 main dish servings; 4 appetizer servings)

2 tablespoons unsweetened coconut milk

1/2 teaspoon sugar

2 garlic cloves, finely minced

1/2 teaspoon curry powder

1/2 teaspoon cornstarch

1 tablespoon fish sauce or 1/4 teaspoon salt

1 tablespoon lime juice

1 teaspoon oil

8 ounces tender beef sirloin, cut into 1-inch x 2-inch strips

8 bamboo skewers, soaked in water for at least 10 minutes

Thai Peanut Sauce (see below)

1. In a large bowl, mix together coconut milk, sugar, garlic, curry powder, cornstarch, fish sauce or salt, lime juice, and oil. Marinate beef in this mixture for 20 minutes.

2. Thread marinated beef onto skewers. Place beef skewers on the grill and cook them, turning and brushing them occasionally with the marinade, about 3 minutes. If grilling indoors under oven broiler, broil for 3 minutes, turning frequently, and brush the meat with the remaining marinade.

To serve: Thai Beef Satay is served with Thai Peanut Sauce (below) and Thai Spicy Cucumber Salad (p. 64).

Nutrition Information per Serving (as a main dish): 274 calories, 18 g total fat (6 g saturated fat), 75 mg cholesterol, 330 mg sodium, 5 g carbohydrates, 0 g dietary fiber, 23 g protein

Nutrition Information per Serving (as an appetizer): 137 calories, 9 g total fat (3 g saturated fat), 37 mg cholesterol, 165 mg sodium, 3 g carbohydrates, 0 g dietary fiber, 11 g protein

Thai Peanut Sauce

Yield: 1/2 cup (1 tablespoon per serving)

4 tablespoons crunchy peanut butter

2 tablespoons unsweetened coconut milk or 2% milk

1 tablespoon lemon or lime juice

1 tablespoon honey

1 tablespoon soy sauce

1/2 teaspoon oil

1/4 cup water

1 teaspoon ground red pepper or red chile paste (optional)

1. Combine peanut butter, coconut or 2% milk, lemon or lime juice, honey, soy sauce, oil, and water in a small saucepan. Cook over low heat, stirring constantly, until the mixture thickens. For a spicier sauce, add ground red pepper or red chile paste.

To serve: Serve with Thai Chicken Satay (p. 84) and Thai Beef Satay (p. 100).

Nutrition Information per Serving: 60 calories, 4 g total fat (1 g saturated fat), 0 mg cholesterol, 156 mg sodium, 4 g carbohydrates, 1 g dietary fiber, 2 g protein

Korean Beef

(4 servings)

1 pound tender beef sirloin, thinly sliced

3 scallions, finely chopped

2 tablespoons soy sauce

1 teaspoon sesame oil

1/2 tablespoon sugar

1/2 tablespoon honey

2 tablespoons red wine

1/4 teaspoon black pepper

1 teaspoon oil

2 cloves garlic, finely minced

1. Combine scallions, soy sauce, sesame oil, sugar, honey, red wine, and black pepper in a bowl. Add the meat to the mixture and marinate it for 30 minutes.

2. Heat the oil in a frying pan until hot. Sauté garlic until fragrant. Over medium heat, add marinated meat–soy sauce mixture and stir-fry for about 3 minutes.

To serve: Serve hot with Asian Plain Rice (p. 36) and Korean Kimchee (p. 54).

Nutrition Information per Serving: 281 calories, 17 g total fat (6 g saturated fat), 75 mg cholesterol, 523 mg sodium, 5 g carbohydrates, 0 g dietary fiber, 23 g protein

Vietnamese Beef and Bean Sprouts
(2 servings)

1/2 pound tender beef sirloin, thinly sliced
1/2 teaspoon cornstarch
1/2 teaspoon salt
1/3 teaspoon pepper
1/3 teaspoon sugar
2 tablespoons oyster sauce (divided)
1 tablespoon oil
2 garlic cloves, minced
1 small onion, coarsely chopped
2 scallions, cut into 3-inch lengths
2 cups bean sprouts
freshly ground black pepper, to taste

Garnish:
2 sprigs cilantro

1. In a large bowl, combine the beef, cornstarch, salt, pepper, sugar, and 1 tablespoon oyster sauce and marinate for 10 minutes.

2. Heat oil until hot in a large frying pan and stir-fry garlic, onion, and scallions until fragrant, about 1 minute. Stir in marinated beef and stir-fry for 3 minutes. Add bean sprouts and the remaining 1 tablespoon of oyster sauce and toss quickly. Remove immediately from heat.

To serve: Transfer beef and bean sprouts to a serving dish and garnish with sprigs of cilantro. Sprinkle with ground black pepper and serve with rice.

Nutrition Information per Serving: 354 calories, 22 g total fat (7 g saturated fat), 75 mg cholesterol, 763 mg sodium, 13 g carbohydrates, 3 g dietary fiber, 26 g protein

Thai Basil Beef and Broccoli

(4 servings)

1/2 pound tender beef sirloin
1/2 teaspoon cornstarch
1/2 teaspoon salt
1/3 teaspoon pepper
1/3 teaspoon sugar
1 tablespoon oyster sauce
1 tablespoon oil
2 garlic cloves, minced
2 scallions, cut into 3-inch lengths
1 small onion, coarsely chopped

1/2 pound broccoli florets, cut into
   bite-size pieces and blanched
1 red bell pepper, thinly sliced
1 red or green hot pepper, chopped
2 sprigs basil
2 tablespoons fish sauce
1/3 cup water
freshly ground black pepper,
   to taste

1. Slice beef into thin strips.

2. In a large bowl, mix the beef, cornstarch, salt, pepper, sugar, and oyster sauce. Set aside for 10 minutes.

3. Heat oil until hot in a large frying pan and stir-fry garlic, scallions, and onion until fragrant, about 1 minute. Stir in marinated beef and stir-fry 3 minutes. Add broccoli, red bell pepper, red or green hot pepper, basil leaves, fish sauce, and water and stir-fry another 5 minutes.

To serve: Transfer beef to a serving dish and garnish with sprigs of cilantro. Sprinkle with ground black pepper and serve with rice.

Nutrition Information per Serving: 398 calories, 23 g total fat (7 g saturated fat), 75 mg cholesterol, 1,255 mg sodium, 24 g carbohydrates, 7 g dietary fiber, 28 g protein

Seafood

Vietnamese Bean Thread Noodles and Crabmeat
(2 main dish servings; 4 side dish servings)

5 ounces dry bean thread noodles (cellophane noodles)
1 teaspoon oil
2 garlic cloves, minced
1 small onion, finely chopped
1 cup fresh backfin or lump crabmeat
1 carrot, finely shredded
2 scallions, sliced
1/2 teaspoon sugar
1 tablespoon oyster sauce
1/2 teaspoon salt
1 cup water
freshly ground black pepper

Garnish:
5 sprigs cilantro

1. Soak bean thread noodles in warm water for 20 minutes. Drain and cut them into short segments.

2. Heat oil in a large frying pan and sauté garlic and onion until fragrant. Stir in crabmeat, shredded carrot, sliced scallions, sugar, oyster sauce, and salt and sauté for 5 minutes. Add soaked bean thread and 1 cup water, cover, and simmer for 7 minutes.

To serve: Transfer noodles to a warmed platter, garnish with cilantro, and sprinkle with freshly ground black pepper. Pass Sweet and Sour Fish Sauce (p. 47).

Nutrition Information per Serving (as a main dish): 376 calories, 3 g total fat (1 g saturated fat), 59 mg cholesterol, 833 mg sodium, 72 g carbohydrates, 3 g dietary fiber, 14 g protein

Nutrition Information per Serving (as a side dish): 188 calories, 2 g total fat (0.2 g saturated fat), 30 mg cholesterol, 416 mg sodium, 36 g carbohydrates, 1 g dietary fiber, 7 g protein

Chinese Fish Fillets in Sweet and Sour Lychee Sauce

(4 servings)

1-1/2 pounds fish fillet, cut into bite-size pieces
1/4 teaspoon salt
1/4 teaspoon pepper
1/2 teaspoon flour
1 tablespoon oyster sauce
1-inch piece ginger, peeled and thinly shredded
1 garlic clove, finely minced
1 small onion, chopped
3 scallions, cut into 3-inch lengths
1 tablespoon oil

Sauce:
1 cup lychees, juice drained and reserved
1 cup lychee juice (in addition to the reserved juice)
1/4 cup pineapple juice
1/2 cup warm water
1 tablespoon cornstarch
1 medium tomato, seeded and thinly sliced
3 tablespoons fish sauce or soy sauce
1 teaspoon ground red pepper or red chile paste

Garnish:
5 sprigs cilantro
shredded scallions
freshly ground black pepper

1. Marinate fish in salt, pepper, flour, oyster sauce, and ginger. Set aside 15 minutes.

2. Heat the oil in a large nonstick frying pan. Add garlic, onions, and scallions and stir-fry until fragrant. Add marinated fish and continue to cook, shaking occasionally, until fish is cooked.

3. In a small saucepan, combine pineapple juice, water, lychees, lychee juice, cornstarch, tomato, and fish sauce. Cook over low heat, stirring constantly, until the mixture becomes thick and clear. For a spicier sauce, add ground red pepper or red chile paste.

To serve: Place fish on a serving platter. Pour lychee sauce over fish and garnish with cilantro and shredded scallions. Sprinkle with freshly ground black pepper and serve steaming hot.

Nutrition Information per Serving: 276 calories, 5 g total fat (1 g saturated fat), 63 mg cholesterol, 692 mg sodium, 26 g carbohydrates, 2 g dietary fiber, 32 g protein

Chinese/Vietnamese Steamed Fish in Hoisin Sauce
(6 servings)

1-1/2 pounds sea bass, rockfish, blue fish, or snapper, split, cleaned, and scaled

1/4 teaspoon salt

1/4 teaspoon pepper

1/4 teaspoon sugar

1 tablespoon oyster sauce

2 tablespoons black bean sauce or hoisin sauce

2 tablespoons soy sauce

1 teaspoon oil

2 cloves garlic, finely minced

1-inch piece ginger, peeled and thinly shredded

6 black Chinese mushrooms, soaked about 3 hours, thinly sliced

Garnish:

3 scallions, thinly shredded

5 sprigs cilantro

freshly ground black pepper

1. Wash fish inside and out with salted water. Drain and pat dry with paper towels. Using a sharp knife, make shallow diagonal slashes on both surfaces of the fish.

2. Marinate fish with salt, pepper, sugar, oyster sauce, black bean or hoisin sauce, soy sauce, oil, garlic, and ginger for 10 minutes.

3. Transfer marinated fish to a deep dish and add the sliced mushrooms. Place fish in a steamer over boiling water and steam it for 20 minutes.

To serve: Garnish with shredded scallions and cilantro and sprinkle with freshly ground black pepper. Serve with Asian Plain Rice (p. 36).

Nutrition Information per Serving: 165 calories, 5 g total fat (1 g saturated fat), 77 mg cholesterol, 436 mg sodium, 6 g carbohydrates, 1 g dietary fiber, 22 g protein

Vietnamese Salt and Pepper Shrimp
(2 servings)

20 medium shrimp, unpeeled

2 teaspoons flour

1/2 teaspoon of salt

1/2 teaspoon of pepper

1 tablespoon of oil

3 garlic cloves, minced

1-inch piece ginger, peeled and thinly sliced

4 scallions, cut into 1-inch pieces

freshly ground black pepper

1. Devein shrimp, using a sharp steak knife to cut through the shell, but do not remove the shell. Marinate shrimp in a mixture of the flour, salt, and pepper for 5 minutes.

2. Heat the oil in a nonstick frying pan until hot and stir-fry the garlic and ginger until fragrant. Stir in shrimp and scallion pieces and continue to cook, shaking the frying pan occasionally, about 3 to 5 minutes or until shrimp are pink and cooked through.

To serve: Transfer shrimp to a serving dish and sprinkle with black pepper.

Nutrition Information per Serving: 148 calories, 8 g total fat (1 g saturated fat), 91 mg cholesterol, 674 mg sodium, 6 g carbohydrates, 1 g dietary fiber, 13 g protein

Vietnamese Catfish on Dill

(3 servings; 2 skewers per serving)

2 pounds catfish nuggets, cut into small cubes
1/2 teaspoon salt
1/2 teaspoon pepper
1/2 teaspoon curry powder
1 teaspoon oil
1 medium onion, thinly sliced
2 scallions, cut into 1-inch pieces
6 bamboo skewers, soaked in water for at least 10 minutes
1 bunch fresh dill, cut into 2-inch strips

1. Marinate fish with salt, pepper, and curry powder for 15 minutes. Thread fish cubes onto skewers.

2. Heat oil in a nonstick skillet and cook fish skewers until golden brown, turning carefully to cook on both sides. Transfer fish skewers to a plate. Add onion and scallions and stir-fry about 2 minutes.

3. Heat iron serving platter until hot. Transfer fish skewers onto heated serving platter, bedded with fresh dill. Top with onion and scallions.

To serve: Serve steamy hot with Asian Plain Rice (p. 36) or Rice Vermicelli (p. 98), Garden Salad (p. 65), and Sweet and Sour Fish Sauce (p. 47).

Nutrition Information per Serving: 221 calories, 12g total fat (3 g saturated fat), 71mg cholesterol, 276mg sodium, 3g carbohydrates, 1 g dietary fiber, 24 g protein

Thai Flounder in Spicy Basil Sauce
(4 servings)

2 pounds flounder, split, cleaned, and scaled, but with head and tail intact
3 tablespoons flour
1/4 teaspoon salt
1/4 teaspoon pepper
4 tablespoons oil
Spicy Basil Sauce (see below)

1. Wash fish inside and out with salted water. Drain and pat dry with paper towels. Using a sharp knife, make shallow diagonal slashes on both surfaces of fish.

2. Mix flour, salt, and pepper and coat fish evenly on both sides.

3. In a nonstick frying pan, heat oil over medium heat. Gently slide fish into hot oil and fry until golden brown, turning once, until the meat is bright white and flakes easily.

4. Remove fish from oil and place on paper towel to drain.

5. Prepare Spicy Basil Sauce (p. 112).

To serve: Place fish on a serving platter and pour basil sauce over it before serving. Garnish with shredded scallions, sprinkle with freshly ground black pepper, and serve with Asian Plain Rice (p. 36).

Nutrition Information per Serving (with sauce): 298 calories, 10 g total fat (2 g saturated fat), 82 mg cholesterol, 706 mg sodium, 17 g carbohydrates, 1 g dietary fiber, 34 g protein

Spicy Basil Sauce

(Yields 1 cup; 2 tablespoons per serving)

1 tablespoon cornstarch

1 cup water

1 teaspoon oil

2 garlic cloves, finely minced

6 sprigs basil, finely minced

1 fresh green hot pepper, thinly shredded

2 tablespoons sugar

1 tablespoon oyster sauce

3 tablespoons fish sauce

3 scallions, thinly shredded

freshly ground black pepper

1. In a small bowl, mix the cornstarch and water.

2. Heat oil in a small saucepan, and stir-fry garlic, basil, and hot pepper until fragrant. Stir in cornstarch mixture, sugar, oyster sauce, and fish sauce. Simmer over medium-low heat. Sauce is ready when it is clear and thick.

To serve: Serve with Thai Flounder in Spicy Basil Sauce (p. 111). Thai Eggplant in Spicy Basil Sauce (p. 123).

Nutrition Information per Tablespoon: 15 calories, 0 g total fat (0 g saturated fat), 0 mg cholesterol, 106 mg sodium, 3 g carbohydrates, 0 g dietary fiber, 0 g protein

Vietnamese Caramel Catfish in Clay Pot

(4 servings)

1-1/2 pound catfish fillet, cut into
   3-inch pieces

1/4 teaspoon salt

1/4 teaspoon pepper

3 tablespoons caramel sauce

2 tablespoons oyster sauce

5 tablespoons fish sauce

1 tablespoon oil

2 garlic cloves, finely minced

2 scallions, finely minced

1/2 cup water

freshly ground black pepper

Caramel Sauce:

3 tablespoons sugar

3 tablespoons water

1/4 cup warm water

1. For Caramel Sauce, in a small, nonstick saucepan, combine sugar and 3 tablespoons water. Bring to a boil, then turn heat down to medium low and stir continuously until it turns to caramel brown. Add 1/4 cup warm water and continue stirring until the mixture becomes a brown caramel syrup.

2. Marinate fish in a mixture of salt, pepper, caramel sauce, oyster sauce, fish sauce, oil, garlic, and scallions for 15 minutes.

3. Transfer marinated fish to a clay pot or a medium nonstick saucepan. Add 1/2 cup water. Turn heat to medium low and simmer until the fish turns brownish caramel, about 15 minutes.

To serve: Sprinkle fish with black pepper and serve it steamy hot with Asian Plain Rice (p. 36) paired with a bowl of Vietnamese Vegetarian Hot and Sour Pineapple Soup (p. 126). Add fresh red chile pepper to taste.

Nutrition Information per Serving: 317 calories, 16 g total fat (4 g saturated fat), 80 mg cholesterol, 945 mg sodium, 14 g carbohydrates, 0 g dietary fiber, 27 g protein

Seafood Pad Thai Noodles

(*4 servings*)

8 ounces Thai flat rice noodles

1 tablespoon oil

2 garlic cloves, finely minced

1/2 small onion, chopped

4 ounces chicken breast meat, thinly sliced

10 medium shrimp, peeled and deveined

2 eggs, beaten

1 teaspoon sugar

2 tablespoons fish sauce

2 scallions, coarsely chopped

1/2 cup bean sprouts

1 tablespoon crushed peanuts

lime juice to taste

1/2 teaspoon freshly ground black pepper

1 Soak noodles in cold water for 10 minutes. Drain. In a soup pot, bring two quarts of fresh water to a boil. Add drained noodles and cook at a rolling boil for 7 minutes , stirring occasionally, until noodles are tender.

2. Rinse noodles under cold running water and set aside.

3. Heat oil in a large frying pan and sauté garlic and onion until fragrant. Stir-fry chicken and shrimp about 7 minutes. Add beaten eggs, sugar, fish sauce, scallions, and noodles and toss well for 5 minutes over medium heat.

To serve: Transfer noodle mixture to a serving dish and toss with the bean sprouts. Add lime juice to taste and sprinkle with crushed peanuts and freshly ground black pepper.

Nutrition Information per Serving: 388 calories, 10 g total fat (2 g saturated fat), 153 mg cholesterol, 353 mg sodium, 55 g carbohydrates, 1 g dietary fiber, 19 g protein

Vegetables/Vegetarian Delights

Plain Fried Tofu
(16 pieces; 4 pieces per serving)

2 4-inch x 6-inch blocks hard tofu

1/2 cup oil

1. Cut each block of hard tofu into 8 pieces. Heat 1/2 cup of oil in a nonstick frying pan until hot. Carefully add tofu. Turn heat to medium and cook tofu, turning occasionally to ensure an even golden brown color.

2. Remove tofu from oil and place on a paper towel-covered plate to absorb excess oil.

To serve: Serve by itself as an appetizer with any choice of sauces or as a side dish with vegetables.

Nutrition Information per Serving: 141 calories, 10 g total fat (2 g saturated fat), 0 mg cholesterol, 8 mg sodium, 5g carbohydrates, 2 g dietary fiber, 9 g protein

Vietnamese Steamed Tofu with Scallion Sauté

(4 servings)

2 4-inch x 6-inch blocks hard tofu

2 tablespoons fish sauce or soy sauce

1 tablespoon honey or syrup

2 tablespoons warm water

2 scallions, finely sliced

1 teaspoon olive oil

1. Divide each block of tofu into 8 pieces and place in a shallow bowl. Thoroughly combine the fish or soy sauce, honey or syrup, and warm water until honey is emulsified.

2. Pour the mixture over the tofu, add the scallions and olive oil, and place bowl in a steamer for about 10 minutes. You may heat the tofu in a microwave oven if you wish. Heat for 2 or 3 minutes on high, until steaming hot.

To serve: Serve piping hot with Asian Plain Rice (p. 36), Vietnamese Tomato Rice (p. 37), Asian Brown Rice (p. 41), or Vietnamese Lemon Rice (p. 38).

Nutrition Information per Serving: 269 calories, 15 g total fat (2 g saturated fat), 0 mg cholesterol, 285 mg sodium, 13 g carbohydrates, 4 g dietary fiber, 26 g protein

Indian Vegetarian Curry

(6 servings)

1 4-inch x 6-inch block hard tofu and 1/2 cup oil or 1/2 bag ready-fried tofu (available in Asian grocery stores)
1 teaspoon oil
2 garlic cloves, finely minced
1 stalk lemongrass, finely chopped
1 small onion, coarsely chopped
1 red chile pepper
1 medium eggplant, cut into 1-inch cubes
1 teaspoon salt

1/4 teaspoon crushed red pepper
1 teaspoon sugar
2 teaspoons curry powder
1 tablespoon tomato paste
1 cup water
1/2 cup milk
1/2 cup coconut milk
1/2 pound taro root, cut into 1-inch cubes
1 sweet potato, cut into 1-inch cubes

1. If hard tofu is used, follow the instructions in the recipe for Fried Tofu (p. 115).

2. Heat 1 teaspoon oil in a deep pot and stir-fry garlic, onion, lemongrass and red chile pepper until fragrant. Stir in fried tofu, eggplant, salt, crushed red pepper, sugar, curry powder, and tomato paste, and continue to stir-fry for about five minutes.

3. Stir in water, milk, coconut milk, taro root, and sweet potato. Simmer for 20 minutes.

To serve: This spicy dish is usually served with French bread, Asian Plain Rice (p. 36), or Rice Vermicelli (p. 98).

Nutrition Information per Serving: 143 calories, 5 g total fat (1 g saturated fat), 2 mg cholesterol, 460 mg sodium, 20 g carbohydrates, 4 g dietary fiber, 6 g protein

Vietnamese Spicy Lemongrass Tofu
(6 servings)

2 4-inch x 6-inch blocks hard tofu and 1/2 cup oil or 1 bag ready-fried tofu
   (available in Asian grocery stores)

1 teaspoon oil

2 garlic cloves, finely minced

1/2 small onion, chopped

1 stalk lemongrass, tender portion finely chopped

1 hot red chile pepper, minced

1/2 teaspoon curry

2 tablespoons soy sauce or 1/2 teaspoon salt

1 teaspoon sugar

1. If hard tofu is used, follow the instructions in the recipe for Plain
    Fried Tofu (p. 115).

2. Heat 1 teaspoon of oil in the fry pan and stir-fry the garlic, onion,
    lemongrass, chile pepper, and curry until fragrant. Stir in fried tofu
    and stir-fry about 5 minutes. Add soy sauce or salt and sugar, toss
    1 minute, and remove from heat.

To serve: Serve warm with Asian Plain Rice (p. 36), Asian Brown Rice (p. 41), or Rice
Vermicelli (p. 98). Pass Sweet and Sour Soy Sauce (p. 136).

Nutrition Information per Serving: 116 calories, 8 g total fat (1 g saturated fat), 0 mg cholesterol, 313 mg sodium,
 6 g carbohydrates, 2 g dietary fiber, 7 g protein

Korean Cellophane Noodles with Vegetables
(4 servings)

1 4-inch x 6-inch block hard tofu and 1/2 cup oil or 1/2 bag ready-fried tofu
(available in Asian grocery stores)
6 dried Chinese black mushrooms or 6 fresh white mushrooms
5 ounces dry bean thread noodles (cellophane noodles)
1 tablespoon oil
2 garlic cloves, minced
1 small onion, thinly sliced
1 carrot, finely shredded
1 cup snow peas, thinly sliced
1 green pepper, coarsely sliced
1/2 teaspoon sugar
1/2 teaspoon salt
1 tablespoon soy sauce
1 teaspoon sesame oil
1 cup water
1 tablespoon roasted, unsalted sesame seeds
2 scallions, thinly sliced
1/2 teaspoon freshly ground black pepper
Sweet and Sour Soy Sauce (p. 136)

Garnish:
5 sprigs cilantro

1. If using Chinese dried mushrooms, soak them in hot water for
    3 hours, trim hard stems, and pat dry.

2. If hard tofu is used, follow instructions in the recipe for Plain Fried
    Tofu (p. 115). Cut tofu into thin, bite-size pieces.

3. Soak cellophane noodles in warm water for 20 minutes. Drain and cut the noodles into short segments.

4. Heat the oil a large frying pan and sauté the garlic and onion until fragrant. Stir in tofu, mushrooms, carrot, snow peas, green pepper, sugar, salt, soy sauce, and sesame oil and sauté for 5 minutes. Add soaked noodles and 1 cup of water and simmer for 7 minutes. Add sesame seeds and scallions and toss well 1 more minute. Sprinkle with freshly ground black pepper.

To serve: Transfer noodles to warmed platter and garnish with cilantro. Pass Sweet and Sour Soy Sauce (p. 136).

Nutrition Information per Serving: 232 calories, 6 g total fat (1 g saturated fat), 0 mg cholesterol, 536 mg sodium, 43 g carbohydrates, 3 g dietary fiber, 3 g protein

Korean Sesame Spinach or Watercress
(2 servings)

1 pound spinach or watercress
pinch of salt
1/2 teaspoon olive oil
1/8 teaspoon salt
1 tablespoon roasted, unsalted sesame seeds
Vinegar Salad Dressing optional (p. 57)

1. Wash spinach or watercress leaves thoroughly and discard tough stems. Cut leaves in two. Bring a pot of water to a boil, add a pinch of salt, and blanch the spinach or watercress about 1 minute. Rinse in cold water and press down on leaves to expel water.

2. In a mixing bowl, toss spinach or watercress, olive oil, remaining salt, and sesame seeds. Keep refrigerated until serving time.

To serve: Sweet and Sour Fish Sauce (p. 47) or Vinegar Salad Dressing (p. 57) will give the Sesame Spinach extra flavor. Serve Sesame Spinach as a side dish for lunch or dinner.

Nutrition Information per Serving Using Spinach: 83 calories, 4 g total fat (1 g saturated fat), 0 mg cholesterol, 399 mg sodium, 9 g carbohydrates, 7 g dietary fiber, 7 g protein

Nutrition Information per Serving Using Watercress: 58 calories, 3 g total fat (1 g saturated fat), 0 mg cholesterol, 313 mg sodium, 4 g carbohydrates, 4 g dietary fiber, 6 g protein

Vietnamese Salt and Pepper Eggplant with Scallion Sauté
(4 servings)

3 medium eggplants

1 tablespoon oil

1 garlic clove, finely minced

3 scallions, thinly sliced

1/2 teaspoon salt

1/2 teaspoon pepper

1. Turn on broiler and broil eggplants about 5 to 7 minutes until soft, turning frequently to avoid burning them. Remove them from the broiler and set aside.

2. In a small saucepan, heat the oil until hot. Sauté the garlic until fragrant, stir in the scallions, and stir-fry for 2 minutes.

3. Remove charred eggplant skin and, using a sharp knife, slit the eggplant open. Sprinkle with salt and pepper.

To serve: Transfer eggplants to a warmed platter, top with scallion sauté, and serve warm.

Nutrition Information per Serving: 123 calories, 4 g total fat (1 g saturated fat), 0 mg cholesterol, 302 mg sodium, 22 g carbohydrates, 9 g dietary fiber, 4 g protein

Thai Eggplant in Spicy Basil Sauce
(4 servings)

3 medium eggplants

1/2 cup Basic Basil Sauce (p. 112)

1. Turn on broiler and broil eggplants until soft, turning frequently to avoid burning. Remove eggplants from broiler and set aside.

2. Remove charred eggplant skin and use a sharp knife to slit eggplant open.

3. Pour basil sauce over the eggplant.

To serve: Serve with Asian Plain Rice (p. 36) or Asian Brown Rice (p. 41).

Nutrition Information per Serving: 110 calories, 1 g total fat (0.2 g saturated fat), 0 mg cholesterol, 151 mg sodium, 25 g carbohydrates, 9 g dietary fiber, 4 g protein

Vegetarian Pad Thai
(4 servings)

8 ounces Thai flat rice noodles

1 4-inch x 6-inch block hard tofu
   and 1/4 cup oil or 1/2 bag ready-
   fried tofu (available in Asian
   grocery stores)

1 tablespoon oil

1 garlic clove, finely minced

1/2 small onion, chopped

2 eggs, beaten

1 teaspoon sugar

2 tablespoons fish sauce or
   soy sauce

2 scallions, coarsely chopped

1/2 cup bean sprouts

1 tablespoon lime juice

1 tablespoon crushed peanuts

1/2 teaspoon freshly ground black
   pepper

Sweet and Sour Soy Sauce (p. 136)
   (optional)

1. Soak noodles in cold water for 10 minutes. Drain. In a soup pot,
   bring two quarts of water to a boil. Add drained noodles and cook
   at a rolling boil for 7 minutes, stirring occasionally, until noodles
   are tender.

2. Rinse noodles under cold running water and set aside.

3. Cut each block of hard tofu into 8 pieces. Heat 1/4 cup oil and sauté
   tofu until golden. Remove fried tofu from pan and drain on paper
   towels.

4. Heat 1 tablespoon of oil in a large frying pan and sauté the garlic
   and onion until fragrant. Stir-fry tofu about 5 minutes. Add beaten
   eggs, sugar, fish or soy sauce, scallions, and noodles and toss well for
   5 minutes over medium heat.

To serve: Transfer noodles to a serving dish and toss with bean sprouts. Add lime juice to taste
and sprinkle with crushed peanuts and black pepper. Pass Sweet and Sour Soy Sauce (p. 136).

Nutrition Information per Serving: 377 calories, 12 g total fat (2 g saturated fat), 106 mg cholesterol, 315 mg sodium,
55 g carbohydrates, 2 g dietary fiber, 12 g protein

Vietnamese Asparagus in Tamarind Sauce
(2 servings)

15 stalks fresh asparagus

3/4 cup warm water

1 tablespoon tamarind pulp

1 teaspoon cornstarch

2 tablespoons sugar

2 tablespoons fish sauce

1 tablespoon oil

1 garlic clove, finely minced

2 scallions, cut into 1-inch lengths

1 tablespoon roasted, unsalted sesame seeds

1. Thoroughly wash and trim the asparagus and cut into 2-inch pieces. In a medium saucepan, bring water to a boil and blanch asparagus for 3 minutes. In a colander, quickly rinse asparagus under cold running water and drain thoroughly.

2. In a small bowl, mix warm water and tamarind pulp. Mash tamarind with a small spoon to extract as much of the juice as possible. Add cornstarch and sugar to tamarind juice and mix. Set aside.

3. Heat oil in a nonstick skillet and sauté the garlic and scallion until fragrant. Stir in asparagus for 2 minutes. Pour in tamarind mixture and fish sauce and toss all ingredients well over low heat until all vegetables are well coated.

To serve: Sprinkle with sesame seeds and serve warm.

Nutrition Information per Serving: 201 calories, 9 g total fat (1 g saturated fat), 0 mg cholesterol, 529 mg sodium, 27 g carbohydrates, 4 g dietary fiber, 4 g protein

Vietnamese Vegetarian Hot and Sour Pineapple Soup

(4 servings)

1/4 cup warm water

1 tablespoon tamarind pulp

1 4-inch x 6-inch block hard tofu
and 1/4 cup oil or 1/2 bag ready-
fried tofu (available in Asian
grocery stores)

1 teaspoon oil

2 garlic cloves, minced

1/2 fresh pineapple, cored and
thinly sliced, or 1 can sugar-free
pineapple chunks

1 teaspoon sugar

3 cups Vegetable Broth (p. 81)

1 tomato, cut into 8 pieces

1/2 teaspoon salt

Garnish:

1 scallion, sliced

5 sprigs rau om or culantro, finely
chopped

red chile pepper, thinly sliced

1. In a small bowl, mix warm water and tamarind pulp. Mash tamarind with a small spoon to extract as much of the juice as possible. Set aside.

2. Cut each block of hard tofu into 8 pieces. Heat 1/4 cup oil and sauté tofu until golden. Remove fried tofu from pan and drain on paper towels.

3. In a small soup pot, heat 1 teaspoon of oil and sauté the garlic until brown. Stir in the pineapple and sugar. Add three cups of Vegetable Broth and bring to a boil. Add tamarind sauce, fried tofu, tomato, and salt. Skim off foam and simmer for 5 minutes.

To serve: Garnish with scallions, rau om, and red chile pepper. Serve with Asian Plain Rice (p. 36), Asian Brown Rice (p. 41), or Rice Vermicelli (p. 98).

Nutrition Information per Serving: 159 calories, 7 g total fat (1 g saturated fat), 0 mg cholesterol, 476 mg sodium, 22 g carbohydrates, 4 g dietary fiber, 6 g protein

Vegetable Ragout
(6 servings)

1 4-inch x 6-inch block hard tofu and 1/4 cup oil or 1/2 bag
   ready-fried tofu (available in Asian grocery stores)
1 teaspoon salt
1/2 teaspoon sugar
3 tablespoons tomato paste
1 teaspoon oil
2 garlic cloves, minced
1 medium onion, coarsely chopped
4 cups water
1/2 cup red wine
1 medium potato, peeled and cut into large dice
1 cup white mushrooms, cut in half
1/2 cup green peas

1. If hard tofu is used, follow instructions in the recipe for Plain Fried Tofu (p. 115).

2. In a large bowl, thoroughly mix salt, sugar, and tomato paste. Coat tofu with this mixture and marinate for 10 minutes.

3. Heat oil in a deep pot and stir-fry the garlic and onion until fragrant. Sauté tofu about five minutes. Add water and red wine to the pot, stir in the potato, mushrooms, and green peas, and simmer for 20 minutes.

To serve: Serve with Asian Plain Rice (p. 36), Asian Brown Rice, (p. 41), or French bread.

Nutrition Information per Serving: 97 calories, 4 g total fat (1 g saturated fat), 0 mg cholesterol, 461 mg sodium, 10 g carbohydrates, 2 g dietary fiber, 5 g protein

Vietnamese Vegetable Lomein
(*6 servings*)

1 4-inch x 6-inch block hard tofu and 1/4 cup oil or 1/2 bag ready-fried tofu (available in Asian grocery stores)

1 teaspoon oil

1 pound dry egg noodles

1 tablespoon soy sauce

5 dried black Chinese mushrooms or 6 fresh white mushrooms, coarsely cut

2 tablespoons oil

1 small onion, chopped

3 scallions, chopped

1 carrot, thinly sliced

1 cup broccoli, coarsely chopped

1 cup snow peas, coarsely sliced

1/2 teaspoon salt

1/2 teaspoon black pepper

1/4 teaspoon sugar

1 tablespoon oyster sauce or vegetarian oyster sauce

Sweet and Sour Soy Sauce (p. 136)

Garnish:

5 sprigs cilantro

1. If hard tofu is used, follow instructions in the recipe for Plain Fried Tofu (p. 115).

2. Fill a saucepan two-thirds full with water, add 1 teaspoon of oil, and bring to a boil. Add the noodles and cook for 4 minutes, stirring with a fork. Empty noodles into a colander and rinse with cold water. Drain thoroughly. Toss noodles with soy sauce. Set aside.

3. If using Chinese dried mushrooms, soak in warm water for 3 hours or overnight. Cut off hard stems and discard; slice the mushrooms.

4. Heat oil in a large frying pan and stir-fry the onion until fragrant. Stir in tofu, mushrooms, scallions, carrot, broccoli, snow peas, salt, pepper, and sugar, and stir-fry for 2 minutes. Stir in the oyster sauce and remove from heat.

To serve: Place noodles on warmed platter and top with vegetables. Garnish with cilantro and serve with Sweet and Sour Soy Sauce (p. 136).

Nutrition Information per Serving: 410 calories, 12 g total fat (2 g saturated fat), 72 mg cholesterol, 397 mg sodium, 61 g carbohydrates, 4 g dietary fiber, 16 g protein

Thai Tofu and Green Beans in Spicy Basil Sauce
(4 servings)

1 4-inch x 6-inch block hard tofu and 1/4 cup oil or 1/2 bag ready-fried tofu (available in Asian grocery stores)

1/2 teaspoon salt

2 tablespoons fish sauce or soy sauce

1/3 teaspoon pepper

1/2 teaspoon sugar

1 tablespoon oyster sauce

1 tablespoon oil

2 garlic cloves, minced

1 small onion, coarsely chopped

2 scallions, cut into 3-inch lengths

2 cups green beans, cut into 2-inch pieces

1 red bell pepper, coarsely chopped

2 sprigs basil

1 hot green pepper, thinly sliced

freshly ground black pepper, to taste

Garnish:
cilantro sprigs

1. If hard tofu is used, follow instructions in the recipe for Plain Fried Tofu (p. 115).

2. In a large bowl, mix tofu, salt, pepper, sugar, and oyster sauce. Set aside for 10 minutes.

3. Heat oil until hot in a large frying pan and stir-fry the garlic, onion, and scallions until fragrant, about 1 minute. Stir in marinated tofu and stir-fry 2 minutes. Add green beans, red bell pepper, basil leaves, and hot green pepper and stir-fry another 5 minutes.

To serve: Transfer tofu to a serving dish and garnish with sprigs of cilantro. Sprinkle with black pepper and serve with Asian Plain Rice (p. 36).

Nutrition Information per Serving: 151 calories, 9 g total fat (1 g saturated fat), 0 mg cholesterol, 589 mg sodium, 14 g carbohydrates, 4 g dietary fiber, 7 g protein

Stir-Fried Vietnamese Garlic Chives and Tofu
(4 servings)

1 4-inch x 6-inch block hard tofu
1/3 teaspoon salt
1/3 teaspoon pepper
1/3 teaspoon sugar
1 tablespoon vegetarian oyster sauce
1 teaspoon oil
2 garlic cloves, minced
3 scallions, cut into 3-inch lengths
2 cups garlic chives, cut into 2-inch lengths (available in
   Asian grocery stores)
freshly ground black pepper, to taste

1. Drain tofu and slice into 8 pieces measuring roughly 2 inches by
    1-1/2 inches.

2. In a large bowl, mix the tofu, salt, pepper, sugar, and oyster sauce.
    Set aside for 10 minutes.

3. Heat oil in a nonstick frying pan until hot and stir-fry the garlic and
    scallions until fragrant, about 1 minute. Stir in marinated tofu and
    stir-fry gently for 2 minutes. Add garlic chives and stir-fry another 2
    minutes.

To serve: Transfer to a platter and sprinkle with black pepper. Serve with Asian Plain Rice
(p. 36), or Asian Brown Rice (p. 41) and pass the Sweet and Sour Soy Sauce (p. 136).

Nutrition Information per Serving: 141 calories, 8 g total fat (1 g saturated fat), 0 mg cholesterol, 235 mg sodium,
6 g carbohydrates, 3 g dietary fiber, 14 g protein

Garlic Chives and Tofu Soup
(4 servings)

1 4-inch x 6-inch block hard tofu
1 tablespoon vegetarian oyster sauce
3 cups Vegetable Broth (p. 81)
2 cups garlic chives, cut into 2-inch lengths
1/3 teaspoon sugar
1/2 teaspoon salt
freshly ground black pepper, to taste

Garnish:
1 scallion, sliced
5 sprigs cilantro, finely chopped

1. Cut the block of hard tofu into 8 pieces. Marinate tofu with vegetarian oyster sauce.

2. In a small soup pot, bring 3 cups of Vegetable Broth to a boil. Add tofu, garlic chives, sugar, and salt. Skim off foam and simmer for 5 minutes.

To serve: Garnish with scallions and cilantro and sprinkle with black pepper.

Nutrition Information per Serving: 107 calories, 6 g total fat (1 g saturated fat), 0 mg cholesterol, 375 mg sodium, 11 g carbohydrates, 4 g dietary fiber, 6 g protein

Tofu Dip

Yield: 2 cups (1 tablespoon per serving)

1 4-inch x 6-inch block soft tofu, cut into small pieces
1/3 cup fermented tofu
1 tablespoon peanut butter
1 tablespoon vegetarian oyster sauce
1 red pepper, finely minced
1/2 teaspoon black pepper
1/2 teaspoon sugar

1. Combine all of the ingredients and purée them in a food processor.

2. Transfer the tofu purée into a bowl and steam for 10 minutes. Cool and refrigerate.

To serve: Serve as a dip with fresh celery, carrots, broccoli, cauliflower, green bell peppers, cucumbers, or, traditionally, with Garden Salad (p. 65).

Nutrition Information per Tablespoon: 22 calories, 1 g total fat (0.4 g saturated fat), 0 mg cholesterol, 75 mg sodium, 1 g carbohydrates, 0 g dietary fiber, 2 g protein

Vietnamese Vegetable Rolls with Spicy Hoisin Sauce

(8 rolls; 1 roll per serving)

1 teaspoon oil
1/2 cup carrots, shredded
1/2 cup cabbage, shredded
1/4 cup white mushrooms, coarse-
    ly chopped
1/2 medium onion, chopped
1/8 cup crushed peanuts
1 4-inch x 6-inch block hard tofu,
    sliced into thin strips
pinch of salt

1/4 teaspoon pepper
pinch of sugar
4 leaves lettuce (such as romaine)
1 cup bean sprouts
3 mint sprigs
3 basil sprigs
3 cilantro sprigs
8 8-inch round rice papers
Spicy Hoisin Sauce (see below)

1. Heat oil in a frying pan and stir-fry carrots, cabbage, mushrooms, onion, and peanuts until soft. Add tofu, salt, pepper, and sugar. Toss gently and taste for seasoning.

2. Proceed as for Vietnamese Fresh Garden Rolls (p. 43), beginning at instruction number 3.

3. Prepare Spicy Hoisin Sauce (see below).

To serve: Serve with Spicy Hoisin Sauce.

Nutrition Information per Roll: 84 calories, 3 g total fat (0 g saturated fat), 0 mg cholesterol, 196 mg sodium, 12 g carbohydrates, 2 g dietary fiber, 4 g protein

Spicy Hoisin Sauce

Yield: 1/2 cup (1 tablespoon per serving)

2 tablespoons hoisin sauce

1/2 cup warm water

1 teaspoon red chile sauce

1. Mix hoisin sauce and warm water until smooth. Stir in red chile sauce to taste.

Nutrition Information per Serving: 9 Calories, 0 g total fat (0 g saturated fat), 0 mg cholesterol, 65 mg sodium, 2 g carbohydrates, 0 g dietary fiber, 0 g protein

Mixed Vegetables
(4 servings)

1 cup white mushrooms, coarsely chopped
   or 8 dried black Chinese mushrooms
pinch of salt
1 cup snow peas
2 cups broccoli, coarsely chopped
2 carrots, thinly sliced
1 green bell pepper, coarsely chopped
1/2 teaspoon cornstarch
1/2 cup Vegetable Broth (p. 81)
1/4 teaspoon sugar
1 tablespoon oil
2 garlic cloves, finely minced
1 medium onion, coarsely chopped
3 scallions, chopped
3 tablespoons vegetable oyster sauce
freshly ground black pepper, to taste
Sweet and Sour Soy Sauce (see below)

Garnish:
5 sprigs cilantro

1. If using Chinese dried mushrooms, soak them in warm water for 2 hours or overnight. Cut off hard stems and discard; slice the mushrooms.

2. In a medium saucepan, bring water to a boil. Add a pinch of salt and blanch the snow peas, broccoli, carrots, and green bell pepper for about 2 minutes.

3. In a small bowl, mix Vegetable Broth, sugar, and cornstarch.

4. Heat oil in a large frying pan over medium-high heat, add garlic and onion, sauté until fragrant. Stir in scallions and blanched vegetables and stir-fry for 2 minutes. Add cornstarch mixture and oyster sauce and simmer over medium heat until the sauce becomes thick and clear, about 1 minute; and remove from heat.

To serve: Transfer to a serving platter, sprinkle with black pepper, and garnish with cilantro sprigs. Serve with Asian Plain Rice (p. 36) or Asian Brown Rice (p. 41). Pass Sweet and Sour Soy Sauce.

Nutrition Information per Serving: 128 calories, 4 g total fat (1 g saturated fat), 0 mg cholesterol, 143 mg sodium, 22 g carbohydrates, 6 g dietary fiber, 4 g protein

Sweet and Sour Soy Sauce
Yield: 1 cup (2 tablespoons per serving)

2 cloves garlic, finely minced

2 tablespoons sugar

2 tablespoons lemon or lime juice

1/2 cup warm water

7 tablespoons soy sauce

1/2 teaspoon ground red chile pepper, or to taste

1. In a small bowl, mix minced garlic, sugar, lemon or lime juice, water, and soy sauce until sugar has dissolved completely. Add ground red chile pepper as desired.

Nutrition Information per Serving: 23 calories, 0 g total fat (0 g saturated fat), 0 mg cholesterol, 806 mg sodium, 4 g carbohydrates, 0 g dietary fiber, 2 g protein

Desserts

Thai Mango Sticky Rice
(6 servings)

1 cup glutinous rice, soaked for 4 hours
1/2 cup water
1/2 cup coconut milk
1/4 teaspoon salt
1 teaspoon oil
2 ripe mangoes

Coconut Sauce:
1 cup coconut milk
1/2 teaspoon cornstarch
2 tablespoons sugar
1/4 teaspoon salt

1. In a nonstick saucepan, combine rice, water, coconut milk, salt, and oil and bring to a boil. Turn the heat down to medium; stir gently and cook until all water is absorbed. Cover the lid tightly, turn down the heat to very low and cook until rice is done, about 15 to 20 minutes. Before serving, stir rice so it is evenly moist.

2. If you use a steamer, soak the rice overnight and omit the water. Toss rice, coconut milk, salt, and oil in a steamer. Steam for 20 minutes.

3. In a small saucepan, mix coconut milk, cornstarch, sugar, and salt. Cook over medium heat, stirring, until the sauce thickens.

4. Peel the mangoes, slice them lengthwise, and remove the pits. Set aside.

To serve: Divide the rice into 6 plates. Place mango slices on top and pour the Coconut Sauce over the rice.

Nutrition Information per Serving: 156 calories, 1 g total fat (0 g saturated fat), 0 mg cholesterol, 226 mg sodium, 33 g carbohydrates, 2 g dietary fiber, 3 g protein

Chinese Black-Eyed Peas in Ginger and Orange-Flavored Sauce

(6 servings)

1 cup dried black-eyed peas
4 cups water
1 2-inch piece ginger, peeled and smashed
1 cup brown sugar
1/2 teaspoon salt
2 tablespoons orange zest

1. Soak black-eyed peas in plenty of water for at least 4 hours or, preferably, overnight.

2. In a medium saucepan, combine the beans and water. Bring to a boil, then reduce heat to medium low. Stir in smashed ginger and cook 30 minutes. Add orange zest.

3. Stir in sugar and salt, and simmer another 10 minutes.

4. Remove the ginger, and pour the peas into 6 individual bowls.

To serve: May be served warm, room temperature, or cold.

Nutrition Information per Serving: 225 calories, 0 g total fat (0 g saturated fat), 0 mg cholesterol, 203 mg sodium, 51 g carbohydrates, 3 g dietary fiber, 7 g protein

Chinese Soft Tofu in Ginger Sauce

(6 servings)

1 4-inch x 6-inch block soft silky tofu

2 cups brown sugar

3 cups water

2-inch piece ginger, peeled and smashed

1. Cut tofu into bite-size cubes.

2. Mix brown sugar, water, and ginger and simmer over medium heat for about 5 minutes.

To serve: Before serving, warm the brown sugar syrup, add tofu, and simmer 1 minute. Serve warm. If serving cold, add the tofu to the brown sugar syrup and refrigerate for 15 minutes.

Nutrition Information per Serving: 335 calories, 4 g total fat (1 g saturated fat), 0 mg cholesterol, 36 mg sodium, 73 g carbohydrates, 0 g dietary fiber, 6 g protein

Vietnamese Banana and Yucca in Coconut Milk

(*6 servings*)

1/4 cup tapioca pearls, soaked in warm water

3 cups water

1 small yucca, peeled and cut into bite-size pieces (yields 1 cup)

3 bananas, cut into chunks

1 cup coconut milk

1/2 cup sugar

1/2 teaspoon salt

Garnish:

2 tablespoons crushed, unsalted peanuts

1. Place tapioca in a small bowl, cover with warm water, and soak for 5 minutes.

2. In a medium saucepan, combine 3 cups water and yucca. Bring to a boil, turn heat to medium and simmer about 15 minutes until yucca is soft. Stir in banana and tapioca, and simmer another 5 minutes. Add coconut milk, sugar, and salt and simmer another 2 minutes. Remove from heat.

To serve: Transfer 6 individual serving bowls. Sprinkle with crushed peanuts and serve at room temperature.

Nutrition Information per Serving: 195 calories, 0 g total fat (0 g saturated fat), 0 mg cholesterol, 115 mg sodium, 48 g carbohydrates, 2 g dietary fiber, 1 g protein

Yucca Cake
(10 servings)

2 eggs
2/3 cup sugar
1-1/2 cups water
1 cup coconut milk
2 pounds (approximately) yucca, peeled and cut into small pieces
1/4 teaspoon salt
1 tablespoon butter, melted

1. Using an electric mixer on medium speed, blend together the eggs and sugar until smooth.

2. Using a food processor, combine the water, coconut milk, and yucca until the mixture forms a loose paste. Transfer yucca paste into a large mixing bowl and add the egg mixture, salt, and melted butter.

3. Butter a 9-inch-diameter cake pan and line it with wax paper.

4. Preheat the oven to 380 degrees. Transfer the yucca mixture to the cake pan and bake about 1 hour or until golden brown and firm to the touch. Cool on a cake rack at least 2 hours before serving.

To serve: Serve Yucca Cake at room temperature.

Nutrition Information per Serving: 206 calories, 2 g total fat (1 g saturated fat), 46 mg cholesterol, 62 mg sodium, 44 g carbohydrates, 1 g dietary fiber, 2 g protein

Beverages

Vietnamese Fruit Shake

Yield: 2 half-pint servings

1 cup fruit (strawberry, orange, pineapple, or choose your favorites)
1/2 cup 2% milk
1/2 cup water
3 tablespoons sugar
1 cup crushed ice

1. Use blender to mix fruit, milk, water, and sugar on medium speed. Add crushed ice and blend mixture on high speed for 1 minute.

To serve: Transfer to 2 tall glasses and serve immediately.

Nutrition Information per Serving Using Strawberries: 126 calories, 1 g total fat (1 g saturated fat), 5 mg cholesterol, 37 mg sodium, 27 g carbohydrates, 2 g dietary fiber, 2 g protein

Nutrition Information per Serving Using Oranges: 141 calories, 1 g total fat (1 g saturated fat), 5 mg cholesterol, 37 mg sodium, 31 g carbohydrates, 2 g dietary fiber, 3 g protein

Nutrition Information per Serving Using Pineapple: 141 calories, 2 g total fat (1 g saturated fat), 5 mg cholesterol, 37 mg sodium, 31 g carbohydrates, 1 g dietary fiber, 2 g protein

Thai Iced Tea
Yield: 2 glasses

2 bags Chinese black tea or Thai tea or 3 tablespoons loose Chinese or
  Thai black tea
3 cups water
2 pieces star anise
1/3 cup sugar
4 tablespoons half-and-half or evaporated milk or 2% milk
crushed ice

1. In a small saucepan, bring water to a boil. Add the loose tea or tea
    bags and star anise. Simmer for 7 minutes. Remove the tea or tea
    bags, strain, and add sugar. Allow tea to cool and refrigerate until
    serving.

**To serve: Fill two tall glasses with crushed ice and pour in the chilled tea. Top each glass
with 2 tablespoons of the half-and-half or milk.**

Nutrition Information per Serving Using Half-and-Half: 171 calories, 3 g total fat (2 g saturated fat), 15 mg cholesterol,
  26 mg sodium, 35 g carbohydrates, 0 g dietary fiber, 1 g protein

Nutrition Information per Serving Using Evaporated Milk: 171 calories, 2 g total fat (2 g saturated fat), 10 mg cholesterol,
  41 mg sodium, 37 g carbohydrates, 0 g dietary fiber, 2 g protein

Nutrition Information per Serving Using 2% Milk: 146 calories, 1 g total fat (.4 g saturated fat), 2 mg cholesterol,
  26 mg sodium, 35 g carbohydrates, 0 g dietary fiber, 1 g protein

Artichoke Tea

Yield: 7 quarts (28 servings, 1 cup per serving)

8 quarts water

3 whole artichokes, cut in half

1 teaspoon sugar per cup (if you prefer it sweetened)

1. In a large soup pot, combine the water and artichoke and bring to a boil. Simmer about 45 minutes. Remove from heat, strain, and transfer to a pitcher. Refrigerate.

To serve: Serve hot or cold. If serving hot, microwave 1 cup of Artichoke Tea about 20 seconds. Add sugar to taste.

Nutrition Information per Serving without Sugar: 6 calories, 0 g total fat (0 g saturated fat), 0 mg cholesterol, 20 mg sodium, 1 g carbohydrates, 1 g dietary fiber, 0 g protein

Nutrition Information per Serving with 1 Teaspoon Sugar: 23 calories, 0 g total fat (0 g saturated fat), 0 mg cholesterol, 20 mg sodium, 6 g carbohydrates, 1 g dietary fiber, 0 g protein

Ginger Tea

Yield: 2 cups

1 bag or 1 teaspoon jasmine (or your favorite) tea

2 thin slices ginger

2 cups boiling water

1. Put tea and ginger into a warmed teapot and pour in the boiling water. Let steep about 5 minutes before serving.

Nutrition Information per Serving: 4 calories, 0 g fat (0 g saturated fat), 0 mg cholesterol, 7 mg sodium, 1 g carbohydrates, 0 g dietary fiber, 0 g protein

Soybean Milk

Yield: 3 quarts (12 servings; 1 cup per serving)

3 cups dry soybeans (yields 8 cups of soaked soybeans)
4 quarts water (16 cups)
12-inch x 12-inch clean cheesecloth for straining
1 teaspoon sugar per cup (if you prefer it sweetened)

1. Cover the beans with water and soak overnight. Drain and discard the soaking water.

2. Use the blender to purée the soaked beans—2 cups of soaked soybeans and 4 cups of water at a time. Place a cheesecloth-lined colander over a medium soup pot. Pour the soybean purée into the cloth-lined colander and, using a large spoon, strain out as much liquid as possible from the soybean solids. Discard the solids.

3. Bring the soybean liquid to a boil. Immediately lower the heat and simmer on low for 15 minutes. Remove from heat and allow milk to cool. Pour into a pitcher and keep refrigerated.

To serve: Serve hot or cold. If serving hot, microwave 1 cup of soybean milk for about 30 seconds. Serve by itself or add 1 teaspoon of sugar per cup.

Nutrition Information per Serving without Sugar: 193 calories, 9 g total fat (1 g saturated fat), 0 mg cholesterol, 8 mg sodium, 14 g carbohydrates, 4 g dietary fiber, 17 g protein

Nutrition Information per Serving with Sugar: 210 calories, 9 g total fat (1 g saturated fat), 0 mg cholesterol, 8 mg sodium, 18 g carbohydrates, 4 g dietary fiber, 17 g protein

PART 3

Staying Slim

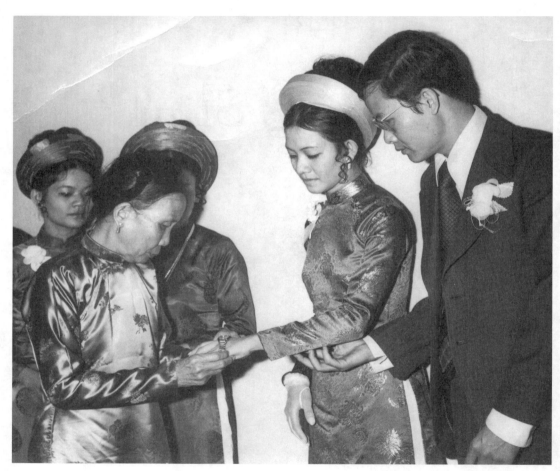

Married at 18, I never thought of worrying about my weight. Living in America, with the introduction of a Western culture, I have to pay more attention to foods and exercise. Being active and eating traditional food helps to keep me healthy and maintain my size.

5 A Maintenance Plan

Once you've lost the weight you want, what comes next? How do you maintain that loss?

First Things First

The first thing you have to do after following a weight loss plan is to add calories slowly back to a level where you can maintain your weight. You do this by adding 100 calories to your plan for two weeks, then checking your weight. If you are still losing weight, add another 100 calories for two weeks and check again. This means that, if you were eating 1,400 calories a day to lose weight, the first level you would try is 1,500 calories. If you are still losing at 1,500 calories after two weeks, go to 1,600 calories. Once your weight has stabilized, you know the level of calories you need to maintain your weight. You can add 100 calories by adding a snack (a piece of fruit or a slice of bread or a glass of skim milk will get you close to 100 calories) or by choosing a higher-calorie recipe in this book.

Be sure you continue physical activity; it isn't just something you do to lose weight. Research on weight maintenance is very clear: those who are able to maintain their weight, incorporate physical activity into their lives. Don't ever think of yourself as sedentary again!

Looking Down the Road

In some ways, losing weight is actually easier than maintaining it (believe it or not). While you're losing weight, people constantly compliment you. You get constant reinforcement for your efforts. Once you've lost weight, the compliments come less often, and you'll meet people who never knew you as a heavier person. You have to look within yourself for further reinforcement. Positive self-talk is crucial. Tell yourself what a good job you're doing and compliment your efforts to incorporate physical activity into your life.

Watch out for some common problems that trap many people who are trying to maintain their weight.

Common Trap Number 1: Kidding Yourself

Certain thoughts can derail your best intentions. Be alert for the following messages that can sabotage your efforts.

- "One time won't hurt me." While it is absolutely true that one exception will probably not cause weight gain, many exceptions do. Don't let exceptions become the rule.
- "Maybe it won't show up on the scale tomorrow if I eat this." This turns weight maintenance into a game, not a way of life. While your weight may not increase overnight, you will have engaged in some self-talk that works against you.
- "I'll make up for this tomorrow." A vicious cycle can begin with this type of thinking. If something comes up tomorrow and you can't follow through, you risk feeling as though you failed. This may lead to the negative notion, "I knew I couldn't do it," which can then lead to eating extra calories. You can easily fall into the trap of eating extra calories and putting off doing something about it. If you have a heavy lunch, eat a lighter dinner. Balance your eating right away, not tomorrow or Monday or next week.

What You Can Do

- Set a limit for yourself and take action when you reach that limit. For example, you may set a five-pound weight gain as your limit, or the way your jeans fit as a limit. As soon as you gain five pounds, or as soon as the jeans don't fit the way you'd like, revert immediately to your weight loss program to lose the weight. Then return to maintenance mode.

- Monitor yourself. If you feel as though your eating is getting out of control, start keeping records of everything you eat and drink for a week. Look critically at what you've consumed and evaluate what you're doing and what you can change.

Common Trap Number 2: Holiday Hazards

There are certain situations that can foil your maintenance attempts if you're not proactive. Holidays, birthdays, and social situations usually include snacking on higher-calorie foods and, sometimes, alcohol. Alcohol not only has calories, it also relaxes your resolve. Once you've had a couple drinks, the benefits of maintaining a lower weight may not be as clear.

What You Can Do

Offer to bring a dish that is lower in calories. If you are the host, plan dishes that fit with your eating plan. Your guests will appreciate the choices. Eat a lighter breakfast and lunch. Don't skip meals, because this may make you ravenous when you reach the party. Dilute your drinks or have one alcoholic beverage and then a seltzer with lemon or lime.

Common Trap Number 3: Down Days

When you feel stressed, depressed, bored, or fatigued, you may be at greater risk for not keeping to your eating and activity plan. You may turn to food to give you that quick boost, or you may pass on your planned activity because you're too tired.

What You Can Do

Make sure you take care of yourself by getting enough sleep. Surround yourself with positive people. Recognize that physical activity can actually increase your energy. Vary your physical activity, and keep records of the type and amount of physical activity you're doing. Add routines or activity types if you find yourself getting bored. Find a buddy, join a gym, learn a new skill—just don't stop!

You're in Charge

You have the power to change the way you live. Eating healthfully and being physically active are positive choices you can make each day. Changing small things can have big results.

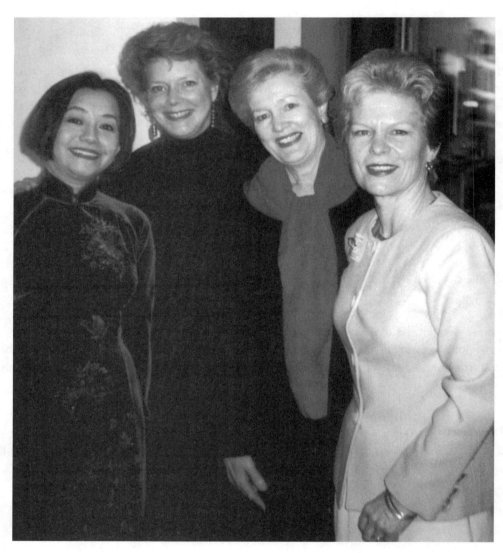

Being in a dressmaking business, I have made many friends. I try every way to "give them a body," whether with the magic of alterations (as my clients state) or with the secret of Asian cooking.

CHAPTER 6

A Nutritionist's Advice

Overweight and Obesity in the United States

More than half of U.S. adults are overweight or obese. The prevalence of obesity has increased steadily over the years, bringing along with it an increase in risk for diabetes, heart disease, stroke, high blood pressure, gallbladder disease, some forms of cancer, osteoarthritis, and sleep apnea.

Why is weight going up? Although scientists have spent many years studying obesity, they have not solved the riddle of what causes it. We do know that there is an imbalance between calories taken in (through food) and calories expended (as activity). Just what makes this system become imbalanced is still somewhat of a mystery. It looks as though the imbalance is caused by a mix of genetics, diet, lifestyle, and the environment. In some cases, psychological factors also play a role. It is becoming clear that many individuals have a genetic susceptibility to become overweight or obese if the conditions are right. Unfortunately, the conditions are becoming more and more right for weight gain.

The Basics

When calories taken in equal calories expended, weight is maintained. When the number of calories taken in exceed the number expended, weight is gained, and when more calories are expended than taken in, weight loss occurs. What has happened to this balancing act in the last decade?

On the "calories in" side, portions are getting bigger. The size of an entrée in most restaurants is huge. Drinks and burgers are "super-sized," and opportunities to snack on convenient, high-calorie items are nonstop. We can eat all day and all night, since many stores are open 24 hours, and we have an endless variety of snack foods.

The "calories out" side has gotten smaller in recent years. We are becoming more and more sedentary. Only 22 percent of U.S. adults get the recommended amount of regular physical activity (five times per week for at least 30 minutes). Our technological advances have helped us burn fewer calories. We have garage door openers, remote controls for the television, snow blowers, leaf blowers, lawn tractors, and the list goes on.

What Are We Doing about the Problem?

It's not as though people are ignoring the problem. Americans spend billions of dollars annually on weight loss products and services. Why aren't these things working? There are many reasons, but one of the major problems is that we approach weight loss in a negative way. I can't tell you how many people I've seen who decide to start with a clean slate on Monday. In their mind, Sunday becomes the last day of freedom, so food intake is unrestricted. Monday morning arrives, and they "go on" a diet that deprives and denies. By the time Friday arrives, they have had it with passing up foods they want and they go "off" the diet. In other words, dieting usually means "doing without," and life revolves around being "on" or "off" a diet.

A Fresh Approach

I believe we've lost the joy of cooking, and we barely take the time to taste our food. I also believe that eating healthfully has gotten a somewhat tarnished image. Confusion reigns in the nutrition world, contradictory recommendations abound, and many "experts" have demonized foods. I think we need a fresh approach to eating healthfully, and that approach is eating Asian.

When I traveled in the Far East, I was stuck by the fact that the only overweight people I saw were the tourists from Western countries. The lack of obesity was most likely due to many factors, including genetics, lack of access to excess, more physical activity, and a different approach to eating. Asian dishes are made with fresh fruits and vegetables. Herbs and spices add intense flavor, and they are low in fat and saturated fat, saving calories and your heart. They can be made quickly, and they use fresh ingredients. Eating Asian can help you not only lose weight but eat more healthfully as well.

What Does Eating Healthfully Mean?

The U.S. government developed a great visual guide for healthy eating, the Food Guide Pyramid, as shown below. Making up the lower, larger parts of the pyramid are three groups: the Bread, Cereal, Rice, Pasta Group; the Vegetable Group; and the Fruit Group. Meat and milk are included in the pyramid, but they are not at the base. As you can see from the picture, we should have fewer servings of meat than vegetables and grains. Finally, fats, oils, and sweets are at the top, illustrating that they should be used sparingly.

The Asian diet fits well with this philosophy. Dishes use abundant vegetables and fruits, and meat is not the centerpiece all the time, but is used in dishes to flavor, not overpower. Sweets and fats are minimized, but not totally absent, ensuring flavorful dishes. Best of all, the entire family can enjoy them. In my mind, there is nothing worse than having to cook separate meals because one family member is "on a diet."

What the Food Guide Pyramid does not communicate well is portion sizes. I've worked with many people who are scared off by the number of servings from the bread, cereal, rice, pasta group and the vegetable group. We are so used to "super-sized" portions that we don't know what a real portion is anymore. For example, one serving from the Bread, Cereal, Rice, Pasta Group is a half-cup of cooked rice or pasta; many restaurants serve three or four times that amount. I've included a table with the portion sizes for each group below.

Food Group	Example of One Serving
bread, cereal, rice, pasta	1 slice of bread; 1 ounce ready-to-eat cereal; 1/2 cup cooked cereal, rice, or pasta
vegetable	1 cup of raw, leafy vegetables; 1/2 cup of other vegetables, cooked or chopped raw; 3/4 cup of vegetable juice
fruit	1 medium piece of fresh fruit; 1/2 cup of chopped, cooked, or canned fruit; 3/4 cup of fruit juice
milk, yogurt, cheese	1 cup of milk or yogurt; 1-1/2 ounces of natural cheese; 2 ounces of processed cheese
meat, poultry, fish, dried beans, eggs, nuts	2–3 ounces of cooked lean meat, poultry, or fish; 1/2 cup cooked dry beans, 1/2 cup tofu, 1 egg, or 2 tablespoons of peanut butter count as 1 ounce of meat

To become familiar with portion sizes, start measuring your food. You might want to put your regular portion on your plate first, and then measure it and see how well you did. You don't need sophisticated equipment; measuring cups and spoons will do. When you buy meat, be sure to check the weight on the package. You may be in for some surprises! After you measure your food for a few days, you'll be able to eyeball amounts easily. To keep yourself on track, measure your food once or twice a month.

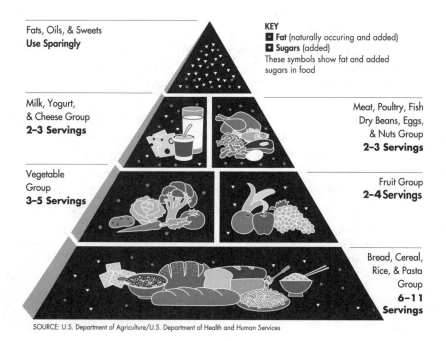

Fats, Oils, & Sweets
Use Sparingly

KEY
■ **Fat** (naturally occuring and added)
▼ **Sugars** (added)
These symbols show fat and added sugars in food

Milk, Yogurt,
& Cheese Group
2–3 Servings

Meat, Poultry, Fish
Dry Beans, Eggs,
& Nuts Group
2–3 Servings

Vegetable
Group
3–5 Servings

Fruit Group
2–4 Servings

Bread, Cereal,
Rice, & Pasta
Group
**6–11
Servings**

SOURCE: U.S. Department of Agriculture/U.S. Department of Health and Human Services

The Process of Losing Weight

Losing weight requires that you take in fewer calories than you expend. This means you have to reduce the number of calories you eat and increase your physical activity. This sounds easy, but if losing weight and keeping it off were effortless, there would not be an obesity problem in this country. Losing weight takes commitment, but it does not require a willingness to eat monotonous, boring food. Where do you start? First, you have to figure out where you are, then plan where you want to be.

1. What should you weigh?

The figure on the next page is taken from the 2000 edition of the Dietary Guidelines for Americans, a government publication. The table shows a range for healthy weight. The lower weights in the healthy weight range apply to women, and the higher weights in the healthy weight range generally apply to men, because women have less muscle and bone than men.

Take a look at the figure and compare your weight to the healthy weight range. Don't think you have to reach a certain number, just use it as a guide. Ask yourself, "At what weight do I feel healthy and good?" Not everyone is born to be extremely slim. The real point is to have the healthiest body you can have, regardless of your shape. Your weight does not tell the whole story about your health. Knowing the amount of

ARE YOU AT A HEALTHY WEIGHT?

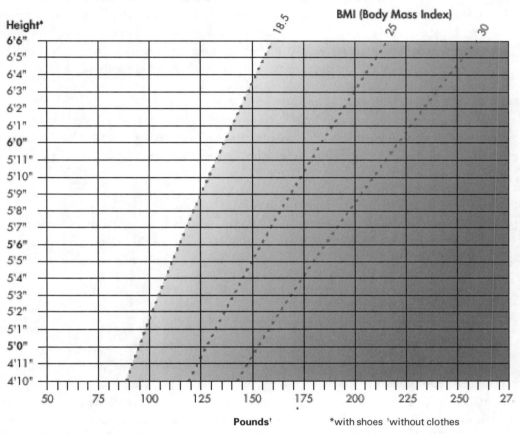

BMI (Body Mass Index)

Height*

Pounds†   *with shoes †without clothes

BMI meaures weight in relation to height. The BMI ranges shown above are for adults. They are not exact ranges of helathy and unhealthy weights. However, they show that health risk increases at higher levels of overweight and obesity. Even within the healthy BMI range, weight gains can carry health risks for adults.

Directions: Find your weight on the bottom of the graph. Go straight up from that point until you came to the line that matches your height. Then look to find your weight group.

Healthy Weight BMI from 18.5 up to 25 refers to healthy weight.
Overweight BMI from 25 up to 30 refers to overweight.
Obese BMI 30 or higher refers to obesity. Obese person are also overweight.

Source: Report of the Dietary Guidelines Advisory Committee on the Dietary Guidelines for Americans, 2000, page 3.

body fat you have and where the fat is located gives you a better idea of how healthy you are. Women have more fat than men because they need it for normal reproductive functioning. For a healthy woman, the optimal range of body fat is 21 percent to 35 percent. For men, the optimal range is 8 percent to 24 percent[1]. Most health clubs

[1] McArdle, W. D., F. I. Katch, and V. L. Katch. *Sports & Exercise Nutrition*. Philadelphia: Lippincott Williams & Wilkins, 1999.

have body fat analysis available, and there are body fat analyzers for home use on the market. More important than the amount of fat you have is where that fat is located. Fat in your abdomen is related to an increased risk of heart disease, high blood pressure, and diabetes. Fat stored in the abdomen gives people an "apple" shape. Women who have a waist circumference of 35 inches or more, and men who have a waist circumference of 40 inches or more, are at higher risk for developing these diseases.

2. How much do you want to lose?

What is the difference between your current weight and your healthy weight? How much of this do you want to lose? Research now shows that for people who are overweight, losing just 5 percent of their weight can reduce the risk of disease, so set a small, realistic goal.

3. What is an appropriate calorie level?

Most women can safely lose weight on 1,200 to 1,400 calories. Most men can lose weight safely on 1,500 to 1,700 calories. Studies have shown that restricting calories too much does not give positive results in the long run. Choose the number of calories that leave you feeling satisfied—not ravenous or stuffed.

4. How long will it take?

Experts advise that you shouldn't lose more than two pounds a week after the first couple of weeks. During the first two weeks or so of a diet, people tend to lose more weight because they are losing water. By about week 3, weight loss should slow to no more than two pounds per week. At this rate, you won't risk your health by losing muscle tissue. Realize that you will hit plateaus—times when you are doing all you can, but the scale isn't moving. We don't know for sure what causes plateaus and we don't know how long they last. Sometimes varying eating and activity routines helps people move beyond plateaus. Recognize that if you are enjoying what you are eating and doing, the plateaus are easier to endure.

5. What else should you do?

- Add physical activity! Experts recommend a mix of aerobic activity and strength training. Aerobic activities, which include walking, swimming, and biking, use the large muscles of the body and increase your fitness, improve heart health, and burn fat. Start small, maybe 10 minutes every other day. Over a period of a month, work up to 30 minutes on most days. You don't have to do the 30 minutes all at once. Your total for the day should equal 30 minutes, so, for example, you can do a 10-minute walk at lunch, a 10-minute walk after arriving home, and a 10-minute walk after dinner.

Strength training means working your muscles against a resistance such as free weights, machines, or your own body. Strength training helps you build your lean body mass (this includes your muscles). Lean body mass is one of the factors that determine your metabolic rate. Having a higher amount of lean body mass means you'll be burning more calories and will make it easier to maintain your weight. Strength training exercises should concentrate on the legs, back, arms, and chest. Try to include strength training in your schedule at least twice a week. To prevent injury, allow a day to recover between sessions.

- Keep records of your activity and your food intake. It's a real boost to see progress over time with physical activity and food records have been shown to help control food intake.

- Enjoy your food—it shouldn't be thought of as "good" or "bad." The key is balance. If one day you have a higher-calorie food, balance it with lower-calorie choices for the rest of the day. Focus on portion size.

- Don't obsess about setbacks. Everyone overeats now and then. How you react to the incident has more of an effect on your progress than what you actually ate. Try to reassure yourself that it is not the end of the world and you are not a failure. Eating healthfully is a learning process that takes time. I've been working in nutrition for more than 20 years, and I'm still learning new things!

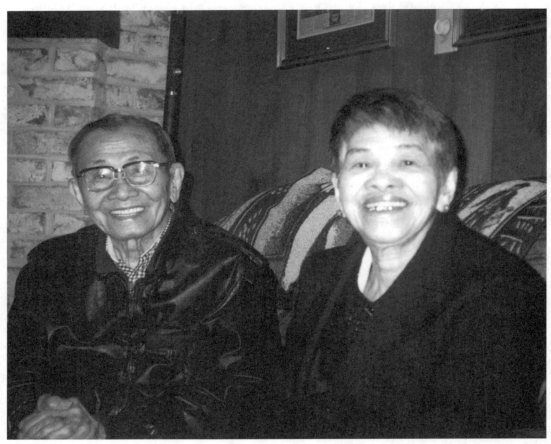

My parents came to America in 1989. Though they try to adapt to American life, they are still very homesick. Cooking is my mother's joy and enjoying her food is my father's interest.

7 A Dressmaker's Advice

I have been in the dressmaking/bridal business, Diana's Couture and Bridal, for more than 20 years. During that time, I have had the privilege of meeting many clients of all races and shapes. In the dressing room, while doing the fitting, we always have a chance to chat. The most interesting subject, or I should say the words that are most often expressed, are "I have gained weight; how can I lose weight and stay in shape?" Frankly, I'm not a doctor or a plastic surgeon, so I can't give them the shape they wish. I can just make the clothes fit right and flatter their figure the best I can with my expertise. Most of the time, I can "get away with murder" and tell them the truth if they have gained a few pounds. Somehow, they tolerate my being too honest. Working mostly with women, my main concern is to make them look good and feel beautiful in their clothes. Because I do fittings, I notice right away any change in their figure, so I can keep tabs on them. Here are some tips:

1. Make a habit of trying on your close-fitting dressy/evening wear once or twice a month. This is a fun way to keep tabs on your shape, and it will either alert you to shape up, if necessary, or to feel good about yourself if you like the shape you see in the mirror. It will also help you build up your self-control and self-esteem.

2. Don't be too intimidated to have your measurements taken every once in a while. I have seen clients come to my store who hate to be measured. Face the truth and try to work on areas that need it instead of avoiding the truth.

3. Set realistic goals when losing weight. One size down at a time is reasonable. Keep in mind that it takes time to lose weight and stay in shape, so be patient.

4. Don't try to wear your clothes too tight or too loose. If they're too tight, they may show flaws, but if they're too loose, they may make you look bigger than you are. While you are in the process of losing weight, it is important to have a few pieces that fit right, preferably separates. Alter your wardrobe gradually as you go along. Seeing your progress is great for your self-esteem.

5. Wear styles and colors that compliment you. Have your colors evaluated professionally. Darker fabrics help to slenderize, and I would prefer plain subtle colors instead of busy prints.

6. Keep up with your looks—when you look good, you'll feel good and vice versa.

Helping Brides and Bridesmaids Lose Weight and Stay Slim

Dealing with brides is really a challenge. Sensitive and nervous, they always expect me to make them the most beautiful bride on their special day. That is quite understandable, but it's not always an easy task. I come up with a plan that I lay out when we first meet. I tell them, "I'll make you a beautiful dream gown, and you'll work on your weight." I try to help them choose the most appropriate design to compliment their body shape. We also discuss their weight goal. If they need time to reach their goal, I am more than happy to give them fittings very close to the wedding date. I also keep tabs on their progress after every fitting and give them a true report on their weight loss. So far, this plan seems to help them control their weight and shape for the wedding date, and it makes my job much easier.

To achieve their goal, I often share with them my Vietnamese diet. I have introduced them to some of the very fast and easy recipes from my first book, *The Vietnamese Cookbook*, published in January 2000. Here I want to share not just the Asian art of cooking, eating well, and staying in shape with little or no effort, but my 20 years' experience in designing and dressmaking as well, to help the bride and her party look their best for the special day.

Your Wedding Gown or Bridesmaid Dress

1. Follow the guidelines in chapter 6. Plan ahead and ask yourself: "If I plan to lose an average of two pounds per week, how many weeks will it take me to reach my goal? Is this in my time line?" Keep in mind that it takes time to get in shape. The more weight you want to lose, the more time it takes. Three to six months is a reasonable span of time to make progress in weight loss. Keep records! Your food record should list the time and the amount of food you eat. Here's an example:

DATE (record the date you start)

Time	Food Eaten
8 a.m.	1/2 cup oatmeal, 1 cup 2% milk, 12 medium strawberries, coffee
12 noon	Vietnamese Chicken Rice Soup Sesame Spinach fresh orange tea
3 p.m.	2 animal cookies, tea
6 p.m.	Asian Brown Rice Chinese Fish Fillets in Sweet and Sour Lychee Sauce Mixed Vegetables Thai Coconut Sticky Rice Artichoke Tea

You also might consider keeping an activity diary, so you can keep track of your physical activity. An example is below:

Date	Time	Activity	Time Spent
Monday, May 5	7 a.m.	walk	10 minutes
	12 noon	walk	10 minutes
	8 p.m.	walk	10 minutes
Tuesday, May 6	6 p.m.	strength training: upper body	20 minutes

2. After you decide how much weight you want to lose, see if it's realistic. If you have a gown custom made, meet with your dressmaker as soon as you can to be measured. Ask for a copy of the measurements to keep on file. Discuss the time the dressmaker needs to work on your dress. Mention your diet plan and how much weight you are trying to lose and ask if the dressmaker can work with you throughout the process. Keep track of your measurements and weight and let the dressmaker know your progress—five to eight pounds make a difference of one to two inches in alteration. The final fitting should be at least two weeks before the wedding date.

3. If you have purchased a gown already, make an appointment to meet with your dressmaker and have the first fitting. Mention your diet plan and ask the dressmaker how much time he or she needs for alterations. Arrange the final fitting and the pick-up date for two weeks before the wedding.

Your Asian Diet Plan

1. Set your weight goal reasonably so that it is workable within your time frame.
2. Use your measurement sheet as a guide. Measure yourself every two weeks. Don't get discouraged—it won't happen overnight!
3. Exercise regularly.
4. Stick with the diet plan. Follow the menu plan and pick the dishes you desire from chapter 4. Of course, every once in a while you can substitute your usual dishes, as long as you stay within the calorie limit. Try to be faithful to it. The foods are enjoyable and it works.
5. Congratulations! You have lost the extra pounds and look great in the gown. Please do not stop exercising and eating right, whether Western-style or Asian. Losing weight for your wedding date is just the first step. Staying in shape, eating healthy, and exercising is your real goal.

Although this chapter is written for brides-to-be and bridesmaids, anyone can benefit from it. Looking good for a special occasion is the greatest incentive to start a diet plan. If you are not a bride-to-be or a bridesmaid, but you do want to lose some extra weight and stay healthy, follow the same diet plan. Pick a special occasion that will give you a strong motivation, like graduation, your birthday party, your family reunion, school reunion, having a new relationship, etc., and start. It may take some getting used to, but I assure you, it will pay off with satisfactory results.

CHAPTER 8

The Joy of Cooking

Looking back on my teen years, I find myself quite amazed when writing this paragraph. I was spoiled by my family; cooking was never my interest. Eating delicious meals, on the other hand, was more my joy. My life suddenly changed the day I left my country to come to Carlisle, Pennsylvania. My homesickness was so overwhelming, I thought I was going to have a breakdown. Happiness came to me through my new beautiful baby boy, sewing, and cooking. To my surprise, I found out that I had some skills. Excited, I tried to replicate the tastes of my homeland I missed so much. I cooked up a storm every day. Somehow, it temporarily took my sadness away.

Cooking became a therapy, a joy that helped me get through the heartache of missing my native land. I realized from that moment on the joy of cooking. My mind was totally involved in the goodness of the foods, the beauty of the finished dishes, and the happiness of my family. At times, I would sing folk songs while washing the vegetables, imagining the happy faces of my family when they tasted my cooking. I felt proud of myself that I could overcome many obstacles.

We moved to Washington, D.C., a year later, where I met Thuy Nguyen, who became my very close friend. We were lonely and homesick together, and we tried to console each other throughout our ordeal. We shared the same experience of the joy of cooking. Cooking, Thuy claimed, is the best way of meditating. It relieves tension and stress after a long day at work. Preparing meals is just like a light exercise for body and mind. During that time, apply a breathing technique, say a prayer, or just concentrate on the beauty of cooking. Cooking can also create family togetherness. It allows parents and children to spend time together and teaches children family values and gives them a sense of sharing, caring, and self-accomplishment. The philosophy is so true that I cannot help mention Thuy and dedicate this chapter to her. She passed away 20 years ago from a car accident, but I will always treasure her philosophy, her joy of cooking, in my heart.

The Recipes

SUBJECT INDEX

Notes

Recipe titles are capitalized (e.g., "Thai Eggplant in Spicy Basil Sauce").
References to photograph insert pages are designated with an italicized
"*P-*" (for example, "staples, *P-1*, *P-3*").

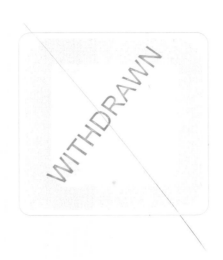